W9-DEE-933

Wellness Coaching for
Lasting Lifestyle Change
2nd Edition

Wellness Coaching for
Lasting Lifestyle Change
2nd Edition

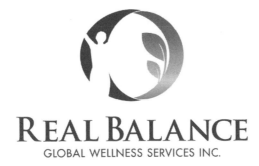

REAL BALANCE
GLOBAL WELLNESS SERVICES INC.

First In Health & Wellness Coach Training

Michael Arloski, Ph.D., PCC, CWP

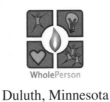

WholePerson

Duluth, Minnesota

Whole Person Associates, Inc.
101 W. 2nd St., Suite 203
Duluth, MN 55802   218-727-0500
E-mail: books@wholeperson.com
Web site: www.wholeperson.com

Wellness Coaching for Lasting Lifestyle Change
2nd Edition
© 2014 Michael Arloski All Rights Reserved

Wellness Coaching for Lasting Lifestyle Change
© 2007, 2009 Michael Arloski All Rights Reserved

No part of this book may be reproduced or transmitted in
any form by any means, electronic or mechanical, including
photocopying, without permission in writing from the
copyright holders.

Reproducible Worksheet Masters and Wellness 360°
Welcome Packet included in *Wellness Coaching for Lasting
Lifestyle Change* are available for purchase on CD from
Whole Person Associates, 101 W. 2nd St., Suite 203, Duluth,
MN 55802, 800-247-6789, www.wholeperson.com.

Printed in the United States of America

Editors: Peg Johnson, Robin McAllister
Art Director: Joy Dey

Library of Congress Control Number: 2014941717
ISBN: 978-1-57025-321-8

WholePerson

101 W. 2nd St, Suite 203
Duluth, MN 55802

Contents

Chapter I

Toward a Psychology of Wellness 1

Chapter 2

Grounded In Wellness: Basic Wellness Principles . . .37

Chapter 6

Creating the Alliance: Let the Coaching Begin!   101

Chapter 7

Charting the Course of Change:
Wellness Mapping 360°™ Part I **123**

Chapter 8

Charting the Course of Change:
Wellness Mapping 360°™ Part II **153**

Chapter 9

Choosing, Living, Loving, Being: Coaching The Strategic, Lifestyle, Interpersonal, and Intrapersonal Aspects of Effective Change. . . 207

Chapter 10

Health and Medical Coaching— Coaching People with Health Challenges 237

Acknowledgements

Through the process of creating this book one concept emerged as paramount in importance . . . connectedness. This book happened because of not only my individual effort, but because of the connections to and with many others. In the present moment my wife, Deborah, has been, and remains a continual support both as my work partner, and my loving life partner. The love and support of family and friends and their continual efforts to maintain connection was also critical through this time.

As I wrote I felt like I was often casting nets back into my past to connect and draw to me learnings that I had experienced earlier and needed to remember now. I acknowledge all those learning gifts that I was given by clients, students, teachers, professors, colleagues, authors, and people I have met around the world.

I am very grateful for the experiences of encounter, gestalt, mind-body awareness and humanistic psychology that I gained at Bowling Green State University from psychologists Melvin Foulds and James Guinan. Those mind and heart-opening experiences helped equip me to connect with others better than I ever had. I also acknowledge a deep gratitude to John Mould, a student of Fritz Perls, my supervisor and mentor for years, who profoundly helped me deepen my psychotherapeutic skills.

Since 1979 I have also enjoyed a sustaining connection that has taken the form of belief in me and my work. John (Jack) Travis and Don Ardell, both pioneers in the wellness field, have continually been there with encouragement, professional stimulation and support. I am also grateful to The National Wellness Institute and Conference, their present staff and board, and their previous directors, Linda Newcomb and Linda Chapin, for their continued belief in me and my work. I also wish to thank Patrick Williams, founder of The Institute For Life Coach Training, for the work we have done together and a wonderful friendship.

Lastly, I acknowledge the shaping and molding that my connections with those I have been especially close to has had over the years. Friends, loved ones, and especially my parents, Anna Merle Arloski, and Joseph John Arloski. I was very fortunate to never doubt their love for even one moment in my life. I dedicate this book to them and their memory.

—Michael Arloski, Ph.D., PCC
November, 2006

Prologue

On the steep hillside where I grew up in eastern Ohio, overlooking the Ohio River, I used to sit on a sandstone boulder and reflect. I would contemplate my young life, and enjoy the shade of the two hundred year old oak tree beside me. Being reflective has been a blessing and a curse all my life, but all in all it has served me well.

In the mid 1970s I began to reflect, as did many of us in the field of behavioral health, on the irony of a nation where the majority of health problems were preventable, and where abundance had spawned our greatest health challenges. We were gathering evidence and awareness that what not only was killing us, but limiting the length and quality of our lives was, in fact, our own choices. All around us we saw health risks being ignored and the consequences being suffered. Obesity, smoking, stress and other factors related to the way we, as a culture, were living were being discovered to be the deadly carriers of our collective "dis-ease".

The fledgling wellness field had begun to grow and capture a lot of excitement and imagination. In 1979 I attended my first National Wellness Conference at the University of Stevens Point, Wisconsin. There I was surrounded by other reflective souls who were not only wondering about these questions of irony and puzzlement, they were implementing ideas of what to do about it! In that wellness milieu I discovered a subculture of like-minded people who were not only studying wellness and lifestyle improvement as an academic subject, they were living it! Living well was, and is, fun!

A flood of health information began to pour forth about our lifestyles and ways to live healthier. You could hardly pick up a magazine or newspaper that didn't have an article about cholesterol or exercise in it. The jogging craze had become the running craze, more young people were backpacking and bicycling than ever before. The public became more and more savvy in the ways of wellness, yet, to our amazement, the health of our nation did not seem to improve that much.

The question for reflection that I have found the most fascinating and the most challenging, is this: *What keeps people from doing what they know they need to do for themselves?* Despite great health information there is still great struggle, for many people, in consistently making the real behavioral changes that create and maintain a healthier lifestyle.

As a behavioral scientist I thought I was a pretty easy teach. Just show me the data that indicates a health risk and I'll believe you and change my behavior to come in line with what is best for my health. Right? Well…that was easy in some areas of my life, and a lot more challenging in others. Exercising and eating right seemed no problem. Taking time to relax, be in nature and spend time with my family…no problem. Get my needs met in the most important intimate relationship in my life…that was a much greater challenge! There is no denying that living well means attending to every area of our lives, especially the ones that are not easy. From my own experience, and the experience of my colleagues, friends, students and clients, I saw that improving one's lifestyle was as much psychology as it was physiology.

My deep interest in biofeedback and behavioral health, as well as Eastern philosophy and spiritual practices, had shown me the potential of our own choices. Through the subtle processes of EEG, EMG and thermal biofeedback, meditative practices, etc., my colleagues and I, in many disciplines, saw how people could exercise influence on parts of the nervous system commonly held to be beyond our conscious control. Through effortless effort people could learn to slow their heart rate, lower their blood pressure, relax their muscles, and even dilate the blood vessels in their extremities. Surely we were discovering, or in some cases re-discovering, new and age-old secrets of how to truly gain conscious control of our lives.

Perhaps some of my interest in approaches that we use in the field of coaching today began in the behavioral medicine and stress-related disorders work that I did for two decades after graduate school. Like coaching, there was an emphasis on awareness, tracking, practicing various relaxation techniques, and reporting in to be held accountable for progress. The results were very measurable, and for the most part, extremely successful!

Clients who had experienced little, if any, success with conventional medicine were finally able to reduce or prevent their headaches, calm their digestive systems, conquer insomnia, minimize anxiety, and more. Central to the approach was educating clients about their challenges (many had no idea how a migraine headache came about or functioned, even after years of treatment) and empowering them to take charge of their own health. Seeing them tap into their own potential for self-regulation was extremely rewarding.

Working with individuals who were motivated to practice relaxation by the positive pay-off of pain reduction, increased sleep, and noticeable improvement in their lives was one thing. Helping people to adopt new behaviors and make it a regular part of their lifestyles was a bigger challenge. When I stepped beyond the treatment-oriented world of behavioral medicine and into the bigger world of wellness, the answers became much more elusive.

Inspired and educated by that 1979 wellness conference, our campus medical director and I brought the wellness concept to Miami University's campus in Oxford, Ohio. We focused on the residence hall system and introduced a health risk assessment and a wellness-environment residence hall program. I began teaching undergrad and graduate classes in wellness and soon began presenting regularly at The National Wellness Conference.

As anyone who works with campus wellness knows, combating the immortality mentality of undergraduates is challenging to say the least! Yet, by inspiring personal growth as well as personal responsibility, and fostering a residential environment with healthy, wellness-oriented norms, we experienced some success.

At the same time my love for the natural world helped me see the connections between lifestyle and environment. I began writing and presenting about the environmental dimension of wellness, helping people see how their own behavioral choices affected not only their own health, but the health of the planet. Contact with the natural world also has a positive effect on our mind, body and spirit. Nancy Rehe and I, at the urging of the president of the Global Tomorrow Coalition, founded a non-profit organization to further these environmental wellness goals.

My attraction to psychology, even as a freshman in college, had always been to the humanistic aspects of the field. The work of Abraham Maslow, Fritz Perls, Carl Rogers, Virginia Satir and others was my earliest draw to wellness as they wrote about self-actualization. In the mid-1990s I discovered that a whole new profession that embraced many of the principles of holism, self-actualization and human potential was developing. The field of personal and professional coaching was getting off the ground and I jumped on board.

Here was an approach to working with people that was about possibilities, not pathology. Here was an approach that held the client to be whole and complete, as they were, right before you. Here was an approach that fostered insight and integration, and then asked the client, "OK, so how can you apply that to your life?"

As I received training in coaching I enjoyed the differences between it and counseling. I saw the value of both, and will always be a powerful advocate of counseling and therapy when it is the method of choice, because I know it works. I deepened my work in coaching and became the Director of Wellness Coaching for The Institute For Life Coach Training.

The blending of wellness and coaching was a natural extension of who I am, and who I had become. For all of our efforts at influencing groups to become healthier through influencing their norms, through wellness education, through incentives and promotions, we saw some success, but many in the wellness and healthcare fields felt disappointment.

Today, with the outrageous (but unfortunately accurate) statistics telling us of epidemic levels of obesity, diabetes, heart disease, and more, combined with the once-again increasing costs of healthcare, solutions are desperately sought. Perhaps the time has come to work on wellness one person at a time.

Wellness professionals are not typically educated in all the interpersonal skills that it takes to work one-on-one. Counselors and others who begin training in the field of coaching may be familiar with holistic health, but are usually not aware of the principles and methods of lifestyle change developed by the wellness profession/industry.

Fritz Perls loved to play on the words of Sigmund Freud about dreams. Freud said that dreams were the "royal road to the unconscious." Perls liked to say that dreams were the "royal road to integration." Perhaps our dream here is one of integration. Perhaps our dream is to develop a new profession that integrates the best of wellness and coaching. Perhaps our dream is to develop qualified professionals who can be the allies that people have long needed to make lasting lifestyle behavioral change.

Introduction

Imagine you are a person who is ready to change your life. Imagine that you want to feel fulfilled in some areas that now seem wanting, or even empty. While certain dimensions of your life are satisfying, even rich, others are a source of frustration at best, and increasing illness and loss at worst.

Imagine that you have expended, over the years, great energy to change and to grow. You have succeeded in some areas but other areas feel like boggy swamps where your progress is like walking knee-to thigh-deep in failure, sadness, regret and perhaps even self-loathing.

Others have tried to help. At times you reached out to them and got information and treatment that kept you going. They may have given you all manner of advice and criticism while imploring and cheering you on. All the motivation seemed based on their own agendas for your life. Despite their efforts, and yours to work with them, you once again feel like you are essentially alone and still bogged down in that swamp.

Now imagine that you begin talking with someone who approaches the process of helping you in an entirely different way. They listen to you—truly listen—not just waiting for their turn to talk. You feel they hear and understand you. Rather than stand above you they stand beside you and with you as an ally. Their agenda is your agenda.

This person does not live with you or work with you, they work for you. You employ them to help you find your way through that swamp that impedes your progress. They require you to look into yourself, to acknowledge your strengths and build upon them in order to confront your fears. They ask questions not so much to gain information, as to require you to seek answers from within yourself, to benefit yourself.

They come equipped with tools that help you take stock of your life and with effective methods for change. They acknowledge that you are ready to make those changes and they ask your permission to delve deeper and push you further. You are treated with respect and compassion, while you are confronted and challenged to do your best. When you make a commitment for action, they help you hold yourself accountable so that you will accomplish your goals in the time frame you allocate.

This person goes beyond gathering information and stresses motivation, helping you find within yourself the motivation needed to initiate, sustain and maintain change. They are there to celebrate your success with you. They are your coach.

Lifestyle Change

Over half of what affects your health is your choice of lifestyle. The way you live your life largely determines the level of health with which you get to experience your life. Perhaps this awareness comes slowly, over years of self-awareness and learning about health and wellness and perhaps it comes quickly, in that teachable moment when you receive a diagnosis or in some way encountered a health challenge.

Most of us have had the experience of being diagnosed and treated or have been to a health-educator who implored us to change our lifestyle behavior. This often magnifies our problems and our own sense of failure. These solitary efforts at change are not easy. To quote Pat Williams, the founder of the Institute for Life Coach Training, "If you could have done it by yourself, you probably would have done it by now." There is the growing awareness that people need an ally to work with, and that wellness is a very individual and personal issue.

Worldwide there is tremendous interest in living happier, healthier lifestyles. Wellness products and services are among the fastest growing economic areas. People are fascinated with spas and magazines that promote living a more simple and healthy lifestyle. The popularity of classes in yoga, Pilates, Tai-Chi, and related methods are at an all-time high. Restaurant menus offer more healthy, lower-carbohydrate, lower-fat, and vegetarian options. Paul Zane Pilzer's book *The Wellness Revolution*, calls wellness "the next trillion-dollar industry."

Vigorous in healthier lifestyles is present in spades, but what is really driving our wellness revolution is the phenomenally increasing cost of healthcare. Around the world companies embrace wellness to help with increasing productivity, lowering absenteeism, employee turnover, etc. In the United States where healthcare reform is only beginning, the employer and the employee are both alarmed at how much of their corporate or individual budget goes into the cost of healthcare services and insurance.

Seen as an actual threat to the health of the economy, not just people, reducing healthcare costs has spawned many experiments.

Knowing that amazing amounts of money are lost when patients do not comply with treatment plans disease management firms have proven their worth by providing coaching and coach-like services that improve patient compliance or adherence. We know from the research of the field of Lifestyle Medicine that lifestyle behavior directly affects the course of many illnesses for the better or for the worse. For many years the health promotion field has contended that over half of what affects the health of a population is lifestyle choices. Now is the time for implementing effective ways of changing lifestyle behavior and making it last.

Yet, more and better health information is not enough. Spending a day or a week at a spa, while enjoyable and perhaps even helpful, does not usually effect a lasting change in lifestyle habits. The process of changing human behavior is complex. Slowly, we are looking to those who have studied human behavior, lifestyle and wellness, for the answers. Many effective methods have been discovered and now they need to be implemented so more people can enjoy better lives.

Coaching

The field of personal and professional coaching is well established and continues to grow worldwide. The International Coaching Federation, which sets standards of certification, provides professional development and education in the field, holds annual conferences in the United States, Europe and Australia/Asia. Coaches now work with business executives, managers, small business owners and entrepreneurs, career professionals, artists, parents, students, families, and more to help fulfill a wide variety of missions and objectives. The coach approach has been found valuable not only to one's business and career, but to develop leadership, deepen character, and help people become the architects of healthy, rewarding lives.

Drawing upon the roots of counseling and psychotherapy, management and human development, the coaching profession saw rapid growth in the early 1990s. (For an excellent review see "The History and Evolution of Life Coaching," chapter two, in *Therapist As Life Coach* by Williams and Davis). What evolved was a realization that much of the work being done in coaching was life coaching. Often one's effectiveness and success at work stemmed not from knowing how to do the job better, but from working with the person's belief systems (especially beliefs about themselves), their interpersonal relationships, and their way of living—their lifestyle.

People found that having an ally who could engage them in possibility thinking, hold them accountable to complete their plans and challenge them to be their very best resulted in real growth, real movement, and often, career/business success as well.

As a coaching and wellness professional, I saw the natural fit and the alliance that needed to be created between the fields. It was like knowing two very different people in a small town who cared deeply—passionately—about the same area of interest, but who would walk obliviously past each other day after day. It seemed obvious to everyone else that they would have a great deal to give to each other. I saw the connections and similarity and have worked to introduce wellness to coaching.

Coaching, at its very foundation, is wellness oriented. Coaching holds the client to be a whole individual, responsible for his or her own choices. According to the Coaches Training Institute, "coaching is a powerful alliance designed to forward and enhance the lifelong process of human learning, effectiveness, and fulfillment." Work is done looking at the client's entire life.

As I wrote about wellness coaching and began presenting about the subject, I discovered a few pioneers out there who, like me, had a long-time interest and/or background in health and wellness, and were purposely applying the skills of coaching to helping people with health and lifestyle goals. The fledgling specialty of wellness coaching had taken flight.

Taking Wellness One-On-One

I regularly found myself talking with health educators, nurses, and various wellness professionals who were becoming discouraged at the ineffectiveness of their efforts to help people live more wellness-oriented lifestyles. The nurses would say "I tell them exactly what they need to do, and they (the clients/patients) don't do it!" The health educators would add "We do great programs in health promotion and have wonderful facilities available, yet so many of the people who really need to use the facilities and make changes in their lives never do!"

These wellness professionals also talk about how, increasingly, they were being asked to work individually with employees who were at high health risk. They found that the same prescribe and treat and educate and implore methods they used with large groups showed little or, at best, sporadic success. Their years of professional schooling and training had never included the training in interpersonal skills that are needed when working one-on-one.

Discovering coaching skills, for these professionals, was a true deliverance. Even health professionals whose contact with clients was limited to fifteen minutes at a time found tremendous value in applying the skills of coaching to their work.

Today wellness coaching is finding application in hospitals, clinical practices, company wellness programs, EAPs, insurnce companies, spas and with the individual consumer. In the larger picture there is a shift occurring towards individualizing wellness. Using sophisticated wellness assessments and possessing improved one-on-one skills helps us create realistic wellness plans for individuals. We are better able to serve the health and well being of people who want (and often need) to benefit from lifestyle improvement.

In 2006, Anne Helmke, then with the National Wellness Institute wrote the quote below noting the paradigm shift within the wellness field to embrace coaching. Indeed since I started presenting on the topic of wellness coaching in the late 1990's at The National Wellness Conference we have witnessed a real surge of programs implementing wellness coaching. The same conference now offers an extensive track of wellness programs each year. The shift has already happened!

I think we are on the verge of a major
paradigm shift in promoting health and wellness driven
by coaching. Coaching provides a positive connection—a
supportive relationship—between the coach and the person
who wants to make a change. That connection empowers
the person being coached to recognize and draw on his or
her own innate ability and resources to make lasting
changes for better health and well-being.

—Anne Helmke

Member Services Team Leader,National Wellness Institute, Stevens Point, WI

Mapping The Course

The intention of this book is to create a resource that helps people create lasting lifestyle change through the process of wellness coaching. While there will be some lifestyle improvement information contained in this work, the emphasis is not how to be well, but rather on how to work as a professional ally with people who want to be well.

As in any journey, we want to begin by becoming well-oriented and well-grounded in where we are, who we are, and what we want to do. We will begin with a foundation in some of the best theoretical concepts about how people change their behavior. This is based on the humanistic contributions of Abraham Maslow and adapted to use in wellness coaching.

We will then ground ourselves in an understanding of the wellness principles essential to working with lifestyle improvement. Drawing upon some of the classic contributions of pioneers and leaders in the wellness field will prepare you to venture further into the integration of wellness and coaching.

The trend is moving toward the individualization of wellness and the current models for wellness work are shifting. In applying the coach approach to the wellness field, you will discover a process for taking wellness one-on-one and the benefits of acquiring such skills.

Then it is time to lift your pack, put on your walking shoes, roll up your sleeves and begin your exploration of just what wellness coaching is, what skills are involved, how to learn them, and how to use them. We will thoroughly cover these skills and provide you with tools and resources for further learning and your application of what you have learned.

From this new vista, further down the trail, we'll look out at how the field of wellness coaching is being applied by fellow travelers who are out there contributing to the field and helping people around the world to be well.

This journey doesn't have an "X" on the map where the trail ends, instead, we'll take a good look at what lies ahead and do our best to speculate on what might be around the next bend, or at least, what we'd love to see there.

Happy trails!

Chapter 1

Toward a Psychology of Wellness

If you have built castles in the air your work
need not be lost; that is where they should be.
Now put the foundations under them.

—Henry David Thoreau

The lifework of psychologist Abraham Maslow, was in many ways, the foundation that allowed the concept of wellness to be built. The cornerstone was the posit that human beings have within them an "inner nature" that is continually striving in a positive way to actualize their true potential. Early on in *Toward A Psychology Of Being,* 1962, Maslow outlined principles of self-actualization theory that sound like the predecessors of modern behavioral medicine. He spoke of the importance of encouraging this inner nature, this essential core of the person to guide our lives, thus allowing us to "grow healthy, fruitful, and happy." (p. 4) If denied or suppressed, the lack of expression of this inner nature, he argued, leads to sickness.

Just as we see the striving of individuals towards healthier wellness lifestyles, we see this inner striving for the maximization of potential in action. Even the challenges that people face, in their efforts to be well, are addressed by Maslow. "This inner nature is not strong and overpowering and unmistakable like the instincts of animals. It is weak and delicate and subtle and easily overcome by habit, cultural pressure, and wrong attitudes towards it." (p. 4) When we look at behavioral lifestyle change, the challenges of habit, peer health group norms and cognitive structures resemble closely what Maslow referenced.

So much of the discouragement in people's attempts at lifestyle change could be lessened if we saw the structure inside all of us that cheers on healthy behavior as more delicate and subtle. While he described it as weak, Maslow goes on to say that it "rarely disappears in the normal person—perhaps not even in the sick person. Even though denied, it persists underground forever pressing for actualization." (p. 4)

Inside all of us is this fragile warrior or warrioress for good. Though easily beaten down by greater odds, it always re-emerges to pull us back on course towards health and well-being just as surely as we strive to align our eyes level with the horizon.

Abraham Maslow was not one to deny the realities of this world or sugarcoat our human history. The oldest of seven children born to Russian Jewish parents who immigrated to the United States around the beginning of the twentieth century, Maslow knew a hard life growing up in Brooklyn, New York. Urged by his parents to seek a better life through education, Abraham eventually got his doctorate in psychology. Working under Kurt Goldstein, he was introduced to the concept of self-actualization, which he developed into one of the quintessential theories of human motivation.

Maslow saw that our suffering and challenges serve to bring out greater strengths. He spoke of the "necessity of discipline, deprivation, frustration, pain, and tragedy. To the extent that these experiences reveal and foster and fulfill our inner nature, to that extent they are desirable experiences . . . The person who hasn't conquered, withstood and overcome continues to feel doubtful that he could." (p. 4)

Sometimes called the father of American Humanism, Maslow inspired other famous leaders in psychology to develop therapeutic methods and approaches to self-actualization that founded the human potential movement. People like Carl Rogers, Virginia Satir and Frederick Perls grounded much of their work in Maslow's principals. Much of the groundwork for today's therapeutic, counseling and coaching methodologies are rooted in these contributions.

A key part of the human potential movement was the body-mind or whole-person approach to human behavior. It became more and more apparent that self-actualization was not just an intellectual or cognitive activity. Mind, body, spirit and environment were all considered in the equation that eventually manifested itself in people looking for ways to improve the quality of their lives—their lifestyle.

In the mid to late 1970s all of this combined with increasing evidence and awareness that how we live our lives is a huge determinant of not only our happiness and well-being, but also of our physical health. John W. Travis, M.D. and Don Ardell, Ph.D. began writing about the concept of wellness in ways that helped us all question our lifestyle status quo, and increase our conscious awareness.

In the years since then, we have seen the field of wellness go through a slow, but steady, metamorphosis. The field evolved through focus on health-risk reduction, peer health norms, reducing health-care costs, physical fitness, diet, stress management, and other facets of lifestyle. Wellness has now come full circle, exploring all aspects of being well.

The wellness continuum that Travis developed positions the field of wellness with an eventual goal of self-actualization. As Travis states in *The Wellness Workbook,* 3rd Ed. "The Illness-Wellness Continuum . . . was a melding of the health risk continuum created by Lewis Robbins, MD, MPH (founder of the Health Risk Appraisal) and Abraham Maslow's concept of self-actualization." (Travis, p. xix)

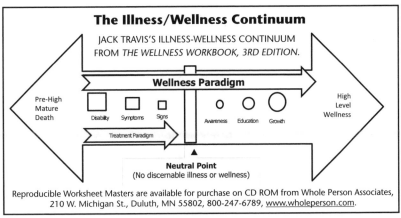

FIGURE 1.1

Don Ardell refers to this as high level wellness and contends, like Travis, that health is not the mere absence of illness, but a continual striving to live a life that is full, meaningful, zestful and exuberant. (Ardell, p. 7)

The eventual goal of wellness is the actualization of one's true psychophysical/spiritual potential. Wellness is Maslow's notion of self-actualization, carried to its natural extension as growth towards the full integration of mind, body, spirit and environment.

This end point is not really an end. It is not perfection. Better than a continuum in this case is a spiral model, continually cycling through the ebb and flow of life towards higher levels of wellness.

Self-actualization is the intrinsic growth of what is already in the organism, or more accurately, of what the organism is.

—Abraham Maslow

Deficiency Needs/Being Needs

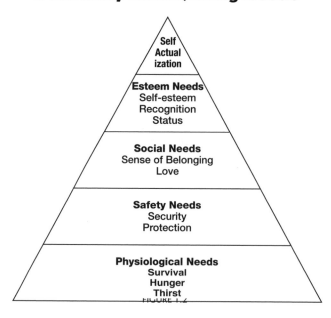

FIGURE 1.2

When we look at Maslow's hierarchy of needs, FIGURE 1.2, through a wellness lens, we see some very familiar terms. Each of his levels of needs correlate with principles most wellness theorists value also.

Maslow's Term	Correlating Wellness Term
Self-actualization	High Level Wellness
Esteem Needs	Adequate Self-esteem
Belonging Needs	Inclusion/Community/Peer Health Norms/Spiritual
Safety Needs	Community/Family/Self-sufficiency
Physiological Needs	Nutrition/Movement/Breathing

FIGURE 1.3

Deficiency Needs

Maslow held that part of being a living organism was that our deficiency needs took precedent in our motivation for behavior. Building from a physiological base, we have to survive and breathing, drinking, and eating always will come first. When deficiency needs are not met we do not function well, and we eventually become ill or die. This applies not only to the obvious situations of suffocation, dehydration and starvation, but also to the somewhat higher (yet still deficiency-based) needs of safety, belongingness, and esteem. When these needs are not met, Maslow argued, we see the rise of psychopathology.

Aberrant behavior and neurosis comes from unmet needs. Using the term illness in both the physical and mental sense he saw a need as a deficiency need, as a basic need or instinct if:

1. Its absence breeds illness
2. Its presence prevents illness
3. Its restoration cures illness
4. Under certain (very complex) free choice situations, it is preferred by the deprived person over other satisfactions
5. It is found to be inactive, at a low ebb, or functionally absent in the healthy person

When we look at the lifestyle of a person we see aspects of it that work their way up through the entire needs triangle. When someone attempts to improve their lifestyle they attempt to meet these needs increasingly effective ways.

Let's use eating as an example.We can eat a very inadequate diet and survive. Sometimes we have to, sometimes it is all we know, and sometimes we know better, yet we eat in ways that don't really serve our health well. The physical need is being met, but, in the long run, how healthy is the way it is being met? Is it really working for us?

Another example would be movement. The human body was born to move! Exercise physiologists and personal trainers will be quick to tell you that it is our lack of movement (or our repetitive isolated and limited movements) that get us in trouble. We literally have a need to move! Our modern world's increasingly sedentary lifestyle is now seen as one of our greatest health risks.

We can take any one of these needs, which all correlate with some dimension of wellness, and overlay them onto the Illness/Wellness Continuum.

When we coach someone towards higher levels of wellness we are, in fact, helping them discover increasingly effective ways of getting their basic needs met. Thomas Leonard, the founder of Coach University and one of the pioneers of the coaching movement, often exhorted coaches to help their clients to do two things: eliminate tolerations from their lives, and meet their needs. Leonard believed that people who acknowledge their wide range of needs and consciously go about meeting them here and now (not waiting until after retirement, etc.), are happier, healthier and more successful.

Being Needs

As renowned lecturer Leo Buscallia reminds us, it's important to be a "human being" instead of a "human doing"! When we feel sated, safe, included, good about ourselves, etc. what is next? Fortunately the field of wellness has long recognized that being truly well is not just about doing OK, or just getting by, but rather, about maximizing human potential.

As seen in Figure 1.3, we can take any dimension of wellness into the realm of being needs where we are engaged in a behavior not just to meet needs, but for higher purposes. We dance because we like to, because it is an expression of who we are. We cast flies to trout, or chuck pork-rind to bass, not just to bring fish home to eat, but for many other reasons, perhaps even to relax to the point where we are actually meditating. (Shhhh! Don't let that secret out!)

Some of our behavior is overtly purposed to explore the spiritual, to transcend our everyday existence, and seek connection with something greater than we are. The monk or nun comes easily to mind, but to one degree or another, this is a realm that we all explore in our own way, in our own time.

Indeed, we see Jack Travis' Wellness Energy System model and Wellness Wheel containing twelve dimensions of wellness, two of them being "Transcending" and "Finding Meaning." Much of the writing of Don Ardell in recent years has focused on the vital nature of finding meaning and purpose in our lives, and how central this is to our own pursuit of higher levels of wellness.

Maslow believed that we naturally seek growth, that it is, given the satiation of the deficiency needs, as powerful as the force that turns barren land eventually into climax forest. This point of view sees humankind as naturally good, and given the right environmental support, continually drawn toward the light.

Keys To Wellness

Maslow was, however, quick to point out that our movement towards growth is not so simple. Here the field of wellness and the field of coaching need to study his writings. If growth is so wonderful what holds people back? What keeps us from progressing smoothly to higher levels of growth and wellness? Why is the growth process often painful?

This is where Maslow reminds us of the power of unmet deficiency needs, "of the attractions of safety and security, of the functions of defense and protection against pain, fear, loss and threat and of the need for courage in order to grow ahead." (p. 46)

Inside us are two sets of forces, one that clings to safety and defensiveness out of fear, and one that urges us towards wholeness and full expression of our true selves.

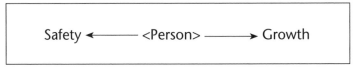

FIGURE 1.4

One part of us is afraid to take chances, afraid to bother the status quo, afraid to move! Another part is driven by a nagging sense of feeling unfulfilled, that our lives will be incomplete unless we express ourselves in some important (to us) way.

In cognitive psychology and in coaching, we often talk about the effect of the inner critic or gremlin on our lives. Here is the continual advocate for safety and the status quo. Here is fear personified, in the sense of the things we say to ourselves that hold us back.

This fear, this need for safety, is not a rational fear—that kind of need for safety we might simply call good judgment. Standing a hundred feet above a lake we might conclude "The cliff is too high above the water, I'm not jumping off!" That is rational fear. The kind of fear our inner critic arouses is based on "**F**alse **E**vidence **A**ppearing **R**eal."

There are certainly attractions to hold to the *status quo*, or even regress when we are under stress. The couch beckons when we are lethargic, not only when we are fatigued. What tastes better than salty, greasy and sweet? Maslow goes on to acknowledge that beyond simple need-reduction there is a hedonic factor. Empty calories taste good!

Knowingly or not, we have been employing some of Maslow's theories in our wellness promotion efforts over the years. When he recommends what we see in Figure 1.5, we can see how this schema has been advocated.

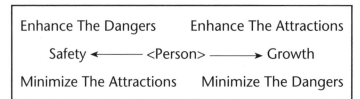

FIGURE 1.5

Health education efforts have exposed the dangers of smoking, sedentary living, etc. Public health efforts have made smoking in public places sometimes inconvenient, and sometimes illegal. We have attempted to enhance the dangers and minimize the attractions of unhealthy behaviors. We have also done our best to make wellness more attractive and appear less dangerous. Yet Maslow says, "safety needs are pre-potent over growth needs." (p. 47)

He notes that "growth forward customarily takes place in little steps, and each step forward is made possible by the feeling of being safe, of operating out into the unknown from a safe home port, of daring because retreat is possible." (p. 47) Yet, what of the outstanding individuals who risk it all, who truly jump from the eagle's nest on untried wings, fall like a stone, and then soar? What conditions need to be present for such risk taking? Of what does that home port need to be composed psychologically?

Being Centered

Let's borrow a metaphor from the martial arts. Perhaps the home port is equivalent to being centered. Being centered is not just a matter of working our internal gyroscope until we are in physical balance. That might be step number one, but there is much more.

When martial artists assume a physically centered stance, they must also center themselves mentally. They do so by focusing on a spot just below the naval, but mid-way between back and belly. They focus on their breath and its rhythm. Their eyes take in their whole field of view at once. On a less conscious but extremely important level they tap into the confidence they have in what they have learned about how to move. They are confident they can move to defend themselves. They feel connected to their vital energy system (the same energy system science has verified through the study of acupuncture, etc.). Their body has been programmed with a set of movements and responses. They know what they can do and have confidence in it. If they are, in fact, a highly skilled martial artist, in the middle of all of this, they are able to relax and move out of conscious awareness.

If they achieve this centered state there is no room for fear. If they let fear creep in, even in the form of expectation of outcome or assumptions of any kind, their probability of remaining safe decreases.

In the much more expansive experience of living our daily lives, rather than meeting a specific physical challenge, how can we apply this notion of being centered, and how do we need to expand it? By exploring what it means for each of us to be centered in our lives we discover what allows us to feel safe enough to grow and move forward towards self-actualization and high-level wellness.

When we consciously seek to meet our needs, when we live our lives in balance, and are true to ourselves, we create that centered life, that safe home port from which to venture out. Clearly much of our most significant growth comes from that venturing out into the unknown. The goal of a life in balance does not mean anxiously attempting to even out everything in our existence. Perhaps living in balance is what allows us to risk, to go the extra mile, to reach summits we never thought we could climb.

The part of us that clings to the safety end of Maslow's continuum can masquerade as a real wellness lifestyle advocate. Under the guise of "balance" it can cause us to walk on eggshells, fearful of not getting enough sleep, of getting hurt or of missing a meal, when the risks are really not that great. Indeed much of our growth comes from experiences on that uncomfortable edge where growth really happens. Real growth may occur when we take the risk of assertively saying no to an unreasonable demand; by pushing through exhaustion and finishing a canoe portage; by steadfastly facing a fear with a loved one; by reaching down deep enough to learn the courage we actually do possess.

Abraham Maslow took on the daunting task of presenting a new theory of human motivation. As challenging as that was, he was up to the task. Here we are considering a less pervasive explanation of human behavior. Perhaps in looking at how can we help people feel safe enough to grow we will find answers to our vexing question about why people don't do what they know they need to do for themselves.

I am convinced that much of what we now call psychology is the study of the tricks we use to avoid the anxiety of absolute novelty by making believe the future will be like the past.

—Abraham Maslow, *Toward A Psychology of Being*

Chapter 2

Grounded In Wellness: Basic Wellness Principles

The concept of total wellness recognizes that our every thought, word and behavior affects our greater health and well-being. And we, in turn, are affected not only emotionally but also physically and spiritually.

—Greg Anderson

There is a maxim that says if you really want to learn something, teach it! I've certainly found this adage to be true. Through the years I have taught graduate and undergraduate courses on wellness, lead workshops and retreats, made presentations on wellness and coaching skills, and taught classes about wellness coaching. I've found it essential to help students of all kinds to begin with a solid foundation in what wellness really is, and I've learned from them what is needed.

There is great confusion and even disparity about what wellness is and what the term means. In my wellness coaching classes I found that most students thought they knew what wellness was—and some did. Others knew a lot about holistic health, but little about wellness. Even the wellness professionals in my classes often lacked some of the basic long-accepted concepts vital to an understanding of wellness.

When I keynoted the ISPA-Europe Conference (International Spa Association) I was amazed to talk with so many people who felt they were working in the center of the wellness field, yet had never heard of many of the authors and organizations that I thought were as central to wellness as Freud is to psychiatry.

A physician at the same conference delivered an excellent Power Point presentation entitled "What is Wellness?" Noting his own incredulity, he showed a slide featuring a German wellness product— Wellness-brand horse hoof balm! Using this balm on the hooves of a horse purported to prevent splitting of the hooves, so I guess that made it a wellness product. Any product that assists a person or an animal to become well can, evidently, be called a wellness product.

Indeed, the toothpaste is out of the tube on defining wellness, and we are never getting it back in. That gives all the more reason to present here some basic principles and concepts that the profession of wellness has developed over the last forty years or so.

What Is Wellness?

The Elusive Definition

In 2004, psychologist Judd Allen, Ph.D., a board member of the National Wellness Institute, surveyed a number of experts in the wellness field to get input regarding a definition of wellness. From that survey he concluded that there appears to be general agreement that:

- Wellness is a conscious, self-directed and evolving process of achieving full potential.
- Wellness is multi-dimensional and holistic (encompassing such factors as lifestyle, mental and spiritual well-being and the environment).
- Wellness is positive and affirming.

It is difficult to differentiate wellness from other disciplines, because wellness can be useful in nearly every human endeavor. Wellness is being applied in related fields, such as health promotion and holistic health. We can assess the degree to which wellness is incorporated into a particular approach or program by asking:

- Does this help people achieve their full potential?

- Does this recognize and address the whole person in all of his or her dimensions?
- Does this affirm and mobilize people's positive qualities and strengths?

Allen stated "We [The National Wellness Institute] have adopted the following definition: Wellness is a process of becoming aware of and making choices toward a more successful existence."

This definition agrees with the input received in the survey's responses from experts in the field of wellness. Some of the survey remarks are below:

- Wellness is a choice, a way of life, a process, an efficient channeling of energy, an integration of mind, body, spirit and a loving acceptance of self. — John Travis

- What are the defining characteristics of wellness? Key components for me include: recognition of the holistic nature of health and wellness; a focus on optimal wellbeing for each individual; attention to and integration of many dimensions of health and wellbeing; individual and community responsibility for 'choosing' to be healthy and the creation and maintenance of healthy environments; and encouraging and supporting others in the pursuit of high-level wellness. Wellness is not focused on the diagnosis and treatment of illness; rather, the goal is helping each individual and community achieve the highest level of health possible. Figuring out how to motivate people to change their behaviors and engage in long-lasting healthy behavior patterns is a crucial and perhaps unique dimension of the wellness effort. — Dennis Elsenrath

- It is a positive approach that implies self motivated action. It implies the application of knowledge and information. Facts alone do not lead to a wellness life. — Bill Hetler

- Being all that you can be. Should we use a phrase that has been worn out by the U.S. Military? Even if it works perfectly? Probably not. Somewhere between self-actualization and Being All That You Can Be must lay a phrase that will say the same thing but be at least somewhat unique. — Irv Moore

- The defining characteristics of a wellness lifestyle/mindset are a strong sense of personal responsibility, exceptional physical fitness due to a disciplined commitment to regular/vigorous exercise and sound diet, a positive outlook and a devotion to and capacity for critical thinking, joy in life and openness to new discoveries about the meaning and purposes of life.—Don Ardell

Wellness is the experience of living life with high levels of awareness, conscious choice, self-acceptance, interconnectedness, love, meaning and purpose. Wellness is the individual's life journey (and our society's larger task) of taking Abraham Maslow's concept of Self-Actualization and applying it to mind, body, spirit and our interconnectedness with other people and our environment.

If you are a wellness professional the confused public may often ask you "So, what is wellness anyway?" You don't have time for a long-winded formal definition. What is your best "elevator speech" definition of wellness? Perhaps the briefest, and most practical definition may be *wellness is living your life consciously in ways that improve your health and well being.*

Conscious awareness is the real cornerstone of living a high-level wellness life. It's realizing that we have a choice. I often teach that a coach's job is remind people that they *have* choices. It's stopping for a moment and making the healthier decision as we hold the restaurant menu. It's remembering that we want to prioritize spending time with friends or our children this weekend instead of just running errands and doing housework the whole time. It could even be working with a wellness coach to consciously co-create a wellness plan to live by.

Defining Wellness Coaching

Psychology is the study of behavior. Psychotherapy is the process of applying the principles of psychology to help people change their behavior. Likewise we might say that wellness is everything about living well in a very conscious way. Wellness programming and wellness coaching are about helping people to improve their lifestyle behavior.

Wellness coaching is a very new field. As it emerges and the world discovers the value of it, it will continue to define and re-define itself. What is clear is that *wellness coaching is the application of the principles and processes of professional life coaching to the goals of lifestyle improvement for higher levels of wellness. It is an alliance between a professional coach and a person (or persons) who, through the benefit of that relationship, seeks lasting, lifestyle behavioral change.*

> *. . . the preventative posture is defensive and largely reactive.*
> *That is, it is designed to protect you against illness or*
> *disease; wellness, on the other hand, achieves the same end*
> *by advocating health enrichment, or health promotion,*
> *and life enhancement.*

—**Don Ardell,** *High Level Wellness*

The Illness/Wellness Continuum

As we saw earlier, the goals of high level wellness and self-actualization are at one end of this continuum, and premature death at the other extreme. There is much more to be gained by a thorough understanding of the Illness/Wellness Continuum.

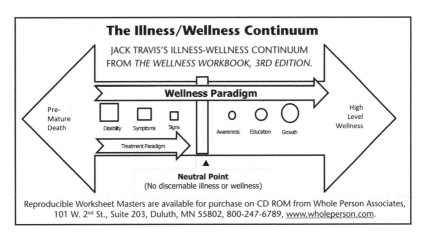

FIGURE 2.1

Wellness is not simply the lack of a disease process or simply the absence of illness. Just as there are degrees of illness, there are degrees of wellness. Wellness, like the way Maslow speaks of self-actualization, is not a static state. It may be counter-theoretical; in fact, to speak in terms of being able to pinpoint one's level of wellness, for it is a fluid, ever-changing process rather than a score or end state.

As we see in the treatment paradigm, however, it is clear that treatment is finished when the person reaches a state of no discernable ill-ness. Treatment is complete and the person usually no longer receives any more services.

Wellness may, at times, actually come into the picture before treat-ment is finished. There is overlap here more than a quick glance at the model might reveal. For example we are finding great benefit in pre- and post-surgical health education, as well as in pre- and post-birth education. The processes of awareness, education, and growth may, in fact, begin before treatment is finished. Among these processes we would include wellness coaching.

Travis and Regina Ryan (co-authors of *The Wellness Workbook*) realized that it is important to also apply the continuum to include those individuals facing health challenges. They readily admit the limitations of a one-dimensional model and now contend that the key factor may not be where a person is physically on the continuum (they could be physically disabled, sick or even in the process of dying), but *which way are they facing.* Are they facing towards high-level wellness with a healthy, positive attitude and a rich spiritual life, or are they facing towards premature death. In this vein, a physically fit marathon winner could be facing premature death, if that person expe-rienced extreme anxiety and strivings for perfection.

Wellness covers the whole continuum. The newly emerging field of lifestyle medicine has extensive evidence that lifestyle very often has a profound affect on the course of an illness. Take for example two people with identical demographic profiles who experience middle-age onset of Type II diabetes. We would place them on the left side of our continuum. Both people are urgently admonished by their health-care team to: quit smoking, lose weight, manage their stress better, be medically compliant and follow their diabetic diet rigorously. Person "A" is successful at all of these challenging lifestyle improvements, while person "B" is not. At the end of two years these behavioral differences result in surprisingly good health for person "A" while person "B" is suffering multiple health problems, has developed co-morbidities, and racked up seriously higher healthcare costs. For both person "A" and "B" wellness mattered.

Wellness and health coaches do, in fact, find themselves working with clients who would fall on the left side of this continuum as much as 80% of the time. Most clients already have either a chronic life-style-related illness, or at least are showing warning signs and conditions such as hypertension or hyperlipidemia. Lifestyle improvement is vital to all.

The good life is a process, not a state of being.
It is a direction not a destination.

—**Carl Rogers,** *On Becoming A Person*

Dimensions of Wellness: Models, Models, Models

The most common misconception about wellness is that it is physical fitness alone, or perhaps physical fitness coupled with nutritional awareness. Diet and exercise/wellness brochures showing pictures of people on treadmills or eating healthy food are mostly what we see.

Wellness (like coaching) is about the whole person and all aspects of their lives. While physical fitness and nutrition are very important, they are only two of the dimensions of wellness. The paradox of any holistic concept is that to be inclusive enough, and to really understand it, we usually have to break it down into its component parts. The gestalt maxim that the whole is greater than the sum of its parts is quite true. Every aspect of our lives affects every other part. An emotional conflict at home will affect our day at work and may even contribute to a headache or some such symptom showing up. An improvement in our diet may result in more sustainable energy all day long, or a better night's sleep.

To ground you in some dimensional models of wellness we have included three of the best known.

Ardell's Model

At the core of Don Ardell's model is *self-responsibility*. As we will explore later in more detail, *you* are primarily responsible for your own health. In his ground-breaking 1977 book, *High Level Wellness: An Alternative to Doctors, Drugs and Disease*, Ardell contends that "The single greatest cause of unhealth in this nation is that most Americans neglect, and surrender to others, responsibility for their own health." (p. 102) Ardell emphasizes that taking personal responsibility for our *choices* is critical in every aspect of our lives. Taking responsibility for our feelings, what we say to ourselves and where we are in our lives is also seen as key to this, and points the way to more effective methods to motivate ourselves to pursue and maintain a more wellness-oriented lifestyle.

The dimensions of physical fitness, stress management and nutritional awareness are forthright enough, but a word needs to be said about environmental sensitivity. The environment in which we live can either enhance or limit our health and well-being. Ardell sees environmental sensitivity as having three aspects: physical, social and personal. This covers many influences in our lives, such as pollution and toxins in our air, water, soil, home and work interiors, and the ergonomics of our workstations.

There are the negative factors that weigh in like noise pollution and heavy metals in drinking water. However there are also ways to affect and interact with our environment to enhance our wellness. Personal growth through contact with the natural world has been the keystone of many organizations developing tomorrow's leaders. From corporate leadership retreats, Outward Bound classes, scouting, and spa nature programs, to spiritual retreats and Native American vision quests, reconnecting with nature is seen as a way to deepen our sense of self and to develop character and purpose. Consciously creating home and work environments that sooth instead of stress the body and mind also contribute to our higher levels of wellness.

Ardell's Model

Self-responsibility
Nutritional Awareness
Stress Management
Physical Fitness
Environmental Sensitivity

FIGURE 2.2

COACHING NOTE

Using Ardell's Model in Wellness Coaching

Ardell's tenet of self-responsibility is a concept key to coaching. My own experience is that until a coaching client accepts responsibility for where they are in their life, including their own health, there is little movement towards improvement. When blame and victimhood are shed, when the client accepts responsibility for his or her own choices, real progress happens. A person may be feeling "stuck" in a job or career that does not serve them well, but when they accept the fact that they have chosen that job or career and they continue to choose to stay with it, they no longer feel trapped by it. A paradoxical sense of freedom emerges and they know they can now make life and health-affirming choices.

This may sound harsh for the person facing particular health challenges, but it applies there too. While one does not "choose" to have diabetes, and there is nothing to be gained by living out one's days regretting all the ways one increased their health risks by years of poor diet and sedentary living, a person can choose the attitude and the way they live with diabetes. Coaching the person with a health challenge requires a thorough exploration of the attitude the client has toward their challenge. The key is helping the client determine what they are responsible for, and helping them to empower themselves to take the action they can for their recovery and the very best life possible. "You are not responsible for your illness. You are responsible for your wellness!"

In coaching you might use Ardell's five dimensions as a way to explore specific areas in a client's life. Stress management, physical fitness and nutritional awareness goals are particularly good candidates. The dimension of environmental sensitivity can be creatively explored and may yield new ideas that help in the other dimensions as well. Increased awareness of one's environment and the effect it has upon one's health can lead to decisions to modify the environment (home improvement, new office lighting, sound proofing, etc.), or even move to a new location. Such decisions can be processed effectively in coaching.

Hetler's Model

Bill Hetler, M.D., Co-founder of The National Wellness Institute developed a comprehensive and inclusive model that looks at wellness in terms of six dimensions:

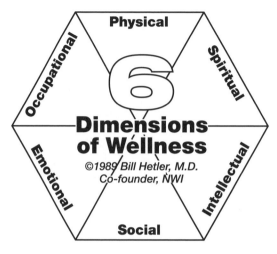

FIGURE 2.3

Since its inception in 1976 Hetler's model has served as one of most common ways to allocate resources for wellness programs. It has been expanded into ten dimensions in TestWell, the assessment instrument developed by the National Wellness Institute (NWI).

1. Physical
2. Sexuality
3. Nutrition
4. Emotional
5. Self Care

6. Intellectual
7. Safety
8. Occupational
9. Environment
10. Spirituality

COACHING NOTE

Using Hetler's Model in Coaching

Wellness coaches may find that using either the six or ten dimensional model of wellness is a very straightforward way to help clients organize their thinking and create a wellness plan that covers each dimension in some way. Using the TestWell instrument as a pre and post instrument (or at intervals during coaching) can serve as a way to stay on track with wellness plan goals. An advantage is that most people can identify what elements of their life fit into each dimension without having to learn any theory.

Travis' Model

In the third edition of The Wellness Workbook (2004), Jack Travis and Regina Ryan elaborate on the Twelve Dimensional Model of wellness that Travis developed. A detailed understanding of each of these dimensions and their interrelationship is best found in the Wellness Workbook itself, but here we will look at some advantages that the model holds for wellness coaches.

Travis' model is based on a theory of energy and energy flow. He sees the dimensions of Eating, Breathing, and Sensing as the way we take energy into the body/mind, and the remaining nine dimensions as ways we transform energy and put it out into the universe.

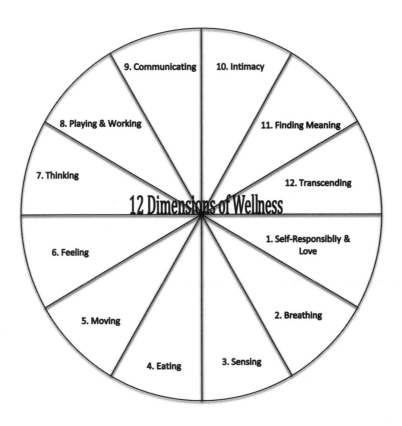

FIGURE 2.4
JOHN W. TRAVIS, MD, MPH 1976, 2004 & HEALTHWORLD ONLINE, INC.

Looking At Each Dimension

1. Self-Responsibility and Love. As a wellness coach you may find your clients make their best progress when they realize they are primarily responsible for their own health. When they take ownership for it they begin to make progress. We look at how loving the person is toward themselves and how connected they feel towards the world around them.

2. Breathing. Coaching about breathing might include not only helping your client to increase their awareness of their own breathing, but also to help them see how easily they are breathing in life. The dimension of breathing looks at the way we either block or allow energy to flow into us, and can be used to help someone find ways to relax.

3. Sensing. Wellness is about conscious living. A great way to increase awareness is through sensory awareness. "Lose your mind, and come to your senses!" is the famous quote by gestalt therapist Fritz Perls. Exploring this dimension can help clients to balance out their intellectual tendencies by becoming more aware of their bodies and what can be learned from them.

4. Eating. There is a distinct advantage to talking with clients about "eating" as opposed to using the trigger word "diet" or "nutrition." This term allows for easy exploration of the role that eating plays in your client's life. Not only is it about what we eat, but how, when, and even why! It can be about how a person digests or takes in their world — what is said to them and what they say to themselves.

5. Moving. When we speak about moving with our clients we avoid the sometimes heavily loaded trigger word exercise. Speaking about movement allows the client to see all their movement in perspective and not just the time they spend working out. Now the client can see such acts as dancing, stair climbing, parking as far away as possible and walking, as movement that can help their health. This expansive notion allows for creative wellness plans that may work where exercise programs have failed before.

6. Feeling. This dimension drives home the fundamental importance of the emotional components of wellness and opens this area up to exploration through coaching.

7. Thinking. This dimension helps clients to understand how thoughts are intertwined and interrelated with feelings and health. Much of the coaching process is about assisting clients to explore the beliefs they hold about themselves and the world. The coach helps clients to examine the thinking that limits them and make new conscious choices.

8. Playing and Working. The coaching process can help clients explore how conscious they are about this dual dimension and how in balance it is for them. A frequent goal of wellness coaching is to increase fun, recreation (re-creation!) and joy in a person's life.

9. Communication. This dimension is a life skill that can either facilitate a smooth journey or bog it down with one conflict or heartache after another. This dimension reminds us that wellness coaching is not just about diet and exercise, but about our ease of connection with others and the integrity of our relationship with ourselves.

10. Intimacy. This dimension allows clients to explore (if they so choose) a dimension of healthy living that is often ignored. Travis takes an approach that sees human sexuality as another form of life energy. There is no judgment here about how it is expressed, but rather an emphasis on flow instead of blockage. The wellness coach, with the client's permission, can help a person explore ways to increase the satisfaction with the way sexuality is expressed in their life. It also helps the client look at the issue of emotional closeness.

11. Finding Meaning. Living a life with meaning and purpose is central to many definitions of wellness. Exploring this dimension can be foundational to making change in any other dimension of living.

12. Transcending. This dimension of wellness may seem esoteric, but it is surprising how often it strikes a respondent chord in clients. The quest to bring one's life into balance by exploring the transcendent side is an ancient endeavor that still speaks to the soul. Again, this dimension can be foundational to other dimensions.

The Iceberg Model of Health and Disease

The Iceberg Model of Health and Disease is a concept that Travis developed that can be helpful in looking at what contributes to the creation of the state of health that is observable. Like the iceberg, we only see the tip of the entire situation. Three-fourths of it lies beneath the surface. Travis sees our state of health as being built upon a foundation of greater and greater breadth and depth. The deepest (therefore the most out of our awareness) and broadest level is what he calls the Spiritual/Being/Meaning Realm. Layered on the spiritual level is the Cultural/Psychological/Motivational Level, and then just below the surface, the Lifestyle/Behavioral Level. Built upon these three subsurface layers is what we see as our state of health.

The Iceberg Model

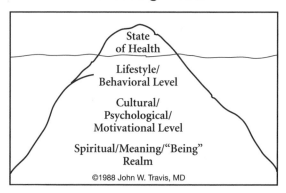

State
of Health

Lifestyle/
Behavioral Level

Cultural/
Psychological/
Motivational Level

Spiritual/Meaning/"Being"
Realm

©1988 John W. Travis, MD

FIGURE 2.5

COACHING NOTE

Using Travis' Model in Coaching

As you coach your client keep in mind that the lifestyle behaviors you and your client are working with have more beneath them. Shifting one's lifestyle without addressing the underlying values, motivations, and philosophical foundations may not allow a person to make a congruent shift and may result in only temporary behavioral change. You may not need to journey to "the depths" with your client for these shifts to occur, but be prepared to help them look deeper into themselves in a variety of ways.

Michael Arloski's Ten Tenets of Wellness

The Encarta World English Dictionary defines a tenet as "any of a set of established and fundamental beliefs." When I originally developed the "Ten Tenets of Wellness" in the early 1990s, I sought not to so much establish a model of wellness, as to set forth fundamental principles of how people can and do change their lifestyle behavior, and what holds them back.

Tenet 1. Wellness is a holistic concept. Anything short of that is incomplete and ultimately ineffective. We need to look at the whole person and create programs (and coach) for the mind, body, spirit, and environment. Just picking the dimension of wellness that you like and minimizing the others doesn't work in the long run.

COACHING NOTE

An exercise in holism

Using "The Wheel of Life" that we referred to earlier, fill in your levels of satisfaction and consider what areas of your life you may have been ignoring. Make a commitment to explore and/or take action in one of those areas in the next week.

Tenet 2. Self-esteem is a critical factor in change. Wellness is caring enough about yourself to take stock of your life, make the necessary changes and find the support to maintain your motivation. Heal the wounds. Find what is holding you back from feeling good about yourself and work through the blocks, not around them.

Everything we do comes either from love or from fear. Where do your wellness lifestyle efforts come from? For many of us, change requires the hard, roll up the sleeves, work of facing our fears and healing old wounds from our experience growing up in our families of origin and our peer group and community. Positive affirmations, or self-statements, are excellent, but need to be coupled with this type of life-long self-reflective work.

COACHING NOTE

An exercise in self-esteem

Identify one negative message you frequently say to yourself ("You're so stupid!" "You'll never amount to anything.," etc.). Relax for a minute or two with your eyes closed. Think of the negative message, and say out loud in a shout "Who says?" Notice who flashes into your mind, a parent, teacher, one-time peer? See with whom you have some unfinished business to deal with.

Tenet 3. Positive peer health norms encourage wellness lifestyle changes. Who we surround ourselves with either helps us stretch our wings and soar, or clips them again and again. Norms are the patterns of behavior that we are surrounded with in our society, our culture, sub-cultures, work-places, neighborhoods, and families. Mutually beneficial relationships with friends, lovers, family and colleagues who care about us as people are what we need to seek and create in our lives. Rather than being threatened by our personal growth, they support it. Do your friends (partners, etc.) bring out your OK or NOT OK feelings? Giving and receiving strokes are what it's all about. Friends keep friends well.

COACHING NOTE

An exercise in positive peer health norms

List who has joined your inner circle of supportive friends in the last ten years. Give thanks, or grieve and get busy making new friends!

Tenet 4. Conscious living means becoming aware of all the choices we have and acting on them. Break out of the trance! Conscious living involves a realization that we don't have to run our lives on automatic pilot. We can turn off the television (remember TV stands for time vacuum), read labels, turn off the lawn sprinklers when we have enough rain, notice how our food tastes, and notice how tense and contracted we are when we drive fifteen mph over the speed limit. Consciously work on relationships, life goals, and maximize our potential.

COACHING NOTE

An exercise in conscious living

For three workdays in a row minimize your attachment to the world of the media. No radio, television, internet, newspaper, or magazines. See what you become aware of about yourself and the world around you.

Tenet 5. A sense of connectedness grounds us in our lives. We are all of one heart. Consciously expanding our web of interconnectedness to other people, other species, the earth and to something greater, may be one of the most powerful acts we can take for being well. Allowing ourselves to move beyond fear and connect with others, to reduce our sense of isolation, can vault us forward in succeeding at lasting lifestyle change. There is a huge difference between **I**-llness and **We**-llness.

Much of this sense of connection can also come out of the land we live on. By identifying with where we live and getting to know the plants, animals, weather patterns, water sources and the landscape itself, we develop not only a love for it, but feel that love returned. Through our commitment to our place on earth we value and protect our environment by the way we live our lives, and by how we speak at the ballot box. Through our contact with the natural world we experience a solid sense of belonging, peace and harmony.

Theologian Matthew Fox likes to say that we can relate to the earth in any of three ways. We can exploit it, recreate on it, or we can be in awe of it. I believe it is within a sense of awe that our potential for growth and healing is multiplied. From such a state of wonder it is easy to see all other species as relatives. The Lakota close every prayer with "Mitakaue Oyasin"—For all my relations.

COACHING NOTE

An exercise in connectedness

Spend twenty minutes in a "natural" area just listening to every sound you hear. Locate origins of the sounds. Identify patterns. Try it with your eyes closed part of the time. Cup your hands behind your ears and try it. Be aware of your responses.

Tenet 6. We are primarily responsible for our health. There are the risk factors of genetics, toxic environments and the like, but our emotional and lifestyle choices determine our health and wellbeing more than anything else. As much as we'd like to cling to blame and copouts, we must be honest with ourselves. The benefit is the empowerment that this realization gives us.

One path out of passivity and illness is to realize what you can do to boost your immune system. Stress, fatigue and poor diet have a tremendous influence on our body's ability to resist illness and disease. Many people report excessive stress and chronic sleep deprivation.

COACHING NOTE

An exercise in health responsibility

To take charge of your own health and boost your immune system, follow the usual wellness advice and live a well-balanced healthy lifestyle but, more specifically, experiment with getting more rest, and practicing some established form of relaxation training.

Tenet 7. Increased self-sufficiency gives the confidence and power that overshadows fear. The Australian aboriginal people say that when a person cannot walk out onto the land and feed, clothe and shelter themselves adequately, a deep primal fear grips their soul. Recognizing our interconnectedness, we grow tremendously when we can care for ourselves on many different levels. Skills, information and tools that enable us to choose our food wisely (or even grow it ourselves); become more competent at our career; adjust the shifter on our bicycle; take a hike into a wilderness area; or bake bread from scratch all increase our self-respect and self-confidence. We need to learn these skills and teach them to others, especially to our children.

COACHING NOTE

An exercise in self-sufficiency

Identify some skill you want to learn that would make your life easier, more economical, or more fun, if you possessed that skill (baking, doing something mechanical, or performing an outdoors skill) Locate a person who you can learn that skill from and arrange an exchange of knowledge, skill, time, or some other way to barter a reciprocal arrangement you both like.

Tenet 8. Time spent alone helps us to get to know ourselves better. As much as we all need time with others, we all need time apart. *Solo time*, especially in the natural world, helps us relax, decontract, and get beyond the distractions of modern life that prevent us from really knowing ourselves. There are some powerful reasons that people from all around the world spend time alone (usually in a wilderness setting) in order to gain vision about the direction and meaning in their lives.

COACHING NOTE

An exercise in solo time

Find a partner who shares your desire to spend one full day in "solo time." Locate a nearby natural area where you both feel safe and where you would enjoy spending the day. Pick a day with a relatively good weather forecast. Take a whistle with you, appropriate clothing, rain-gear, etc. Bring plenty of water, but no food unless you have a special dietary consideration. Do not bring anything to read, or anything with which to write. When you arrive at the area you should both select a small area (a maximum of ten to fifteen yards in diameter) where you would like to spend 5-8 hrs. alone. Your site should be close enough for your partner to hear your whistle easily, but far enough away that you can have complete privacy. Taking opposite sides of the same hilltop ridge works very well for this. Reunite at a prearranged time. Spend your time in contemplation and awareness of everything around you. This is a journey into inner and outer nature. Reflect and write about your experience afterwards if you like.

The goal here is not endurance. Bail out if you have a nasty change in weather or feel ill. You can always reschedule. Though the process of solo time is not physically demanding, you need to be your own judge, or you should seek your physician's advice, if you have health concerns.

Tenet 9. You don't have to be perfect to be well. Extreme perfectionism is a shame-based process that feeds a really negative view of ourselves. Workaholism, anorexia, and other addictive behaviors can result. Wellness does not mean swearing off hot-fudge sundaes. It just means not bs-ing yourself about when you last had one! Whenever our healthy habits move from being positive addictions to being compulsive behavior that works against us, we're usually the last ones to know. Often extreme behavior is a way to distract yourself from some other issue that needs your attention.

COACHING NOTE

An exercise in letting go of perfection

Get a gauge on your diet, exercise and other behaviors. Read several sources and see what the experts recommend. Check your program out with a qualified local resource such as a nutritionist, exercise

> professional or other specialist, then experiment with a free day once a week. If you are the sort of person who can handle it, take one day a week where you give yourself permission to eat anything that you want and medically can have. Remember: ONE day a week!

Tenet 10. Play! We all need to lighten up and not take ourselves (and wellness) too seriously. Remember the lessons of the coyote and be playful, even ornery in a non-malicious way. Let the child within out to play. Give yourself permission.

The work hard, play hard philosophy does little to help us maintain the balance needed for a healthy life. Psychophysiology works twenty four hours a day, every day (not just on weekends). Integrate a healthy sense of humor and play into the workplace. Make sure your yang equals your yin!

COACHING NOTE

An exercise in play

List several of your favorite play activities that you either do, or did at one time in your life. Now, think about when you last engaged in each of these activities. Celebrate or contemplate what you've (temporarily) let go of in your life. Have fun reclaiming it!

Even with these tenets there is no concrete wellness formula. You have to discover what works for you. Take them not as rules, but as modern folklore gathered by one who has walked the wellness way for quite a few years.

COACHING NOTE

Using The Ten Tenets In Coaching

The "Ten Tenets" serve you, the wellness coach, by first of all giving you a fundamental set of principles to help you understand what drives lifestyle change. These tenets attempt to answer the vexing and recurring question "Why don't people do what they know they need to do for themselves?"

Secondly: you can use the tenets as a reference for what you explore in coaching. Ask powerful questions that help your clients consider how well connected they are to their world, how can they feel better about themselves by in some small way becoming more self-sufficient, etc.

Thirdly: you can share the Ten Tenets of Wellness with your client.

Give them a copy of it to read and explore it together. Ask them which of the exercises they might find of value as they explore and experiment within their lives.

You can also attract clients to your coaching by presenting The Ten Tenets and sharing these fundamental principles with your audience. Ask them to identify one or two of the tenets that really seemed to have a message for them in their lives right now.

There are as many reasons for running as there are days in the year, years in my life. But mostly I run because I am an animal and a child, an artist and a saint. So, too, are you. Find your own play, your own self-renewing compulsion, and you will become the person you are meant to be.

–George Sheehan

Chapter 3

Taking Wellness One-On-One:
Changing the Health Promotion Model from Large Groups to Individuals

The People Of The Waterfall, A Folklore Tale

There once was a village of people who lived at the base of a huge waterfall by a lovely river. Life was good until one day a stranger was washed over the falls and plummeted to the rocky cauldron of foaming water beneath it.

The people were alarmed and immediately sent two of their best swimmers out to rescue the person. With much effort the person was dragged ashore and the people succeeded in reviving him.

Before long another stranger was washed over the falls and again a rescue team was sent into the dangerous waters. As they worked on reviving the person they decided to station a rescue boat and a lifeline by the base of the falls.

As time passed, strangers continued to be washed over the waterfall and rescue efforts increased. Soon a small building was erected with emergency supplies and designated people were constantly on call for more rescues.

The number of strangers being washed over the fall continued to increase. Soon the people constructed a small hospital at the base of the falls and built a fine rescue boat with full-time emergency rescue workers to staff it.

The people were perplexed but continued to respond to the demands of the victims of the waterfall. They built an even bigger hospital and started to build a whole fleet of rescue boats, when, at long last, someone asked . . ."Why don't we go upstream and see why these people are falling in?"

Preventive Health

There is obvious wisdom in going upstream and doing something about the source of a problem. In our modern world systems bound to the reactive and remedial are being overwhelmed. Sometimes underfunding keeps the current system on the edge and sometimes the lure of greater financial rewards supports the *status quo*. There is definitely a great deal of money to be made in surgery, pharmaceuticals and other remedial products and services. Prevention is a less profitable area. "Despite spending more than twice what most other industrialized nations spend on health care, the U.S. ranks 24th out of 30 such nations in terms of life expectancy. A major reason for this startling fact is that we spend only 3 percent of our health care dollars on preventing diseases (as opposed to treating them), when 75 percent of our health care costs are related to preventable conditions." Executive Summary, American Public Health Association, June 2012.

We all remember hygiene in our health classes in school. The early days of health education seemed more about cutting those toe-nails in a straight, not curved line than in teaching us about safe sex or how to reduce some more virulent health risks. Although I seem to have had it pounded into my head that a diet composed primarily of highly polished white rice would give me beriberi, I do not remember being taught what a good diet was!

Much of the research that we now take for granted had not been done until the 1970s. Not until the famous Framingham studies of the fifties and sixties did we know that there was a real link between smoking and lung disease, or between our diet and heart disease. Disease avoidance or keeping disease away was the picture of what it meant to be healthy.

In 1961 a little book called *High Level Wellness* was written by Halbert L. Dunn. It was never a bestseller, but it did resonate with a few forward-thinking people in the health-related fields. The revolutionary thing about Dunn's view of health was that he presented it as more than simply the absence of illness. He posited that health and wellbeing were a matter of mind, body and spirit. It was a matter of the whole human being and their personal, social, and physical environment. He described a state of being vitally alive and dubbed it "wellness."

Wellness Full Circle

The field of work that we came to call wellness emerged in the mid-1970's from the body of work by John Travis, Don Ardell, Robert Allen, Bill Hetler and others. They infused the much-neglected area of preventative health with psychological principles of behavioral and development change.

Epidemiology also spurred on some of the first wellness work, largely through the actuarial tables of insurance companies. Cause of death statistics yielded more questions than answers and a great deal of speculation that many factors other than medical were impacting our health.

Studying the relationship between health and behavior yielded the concept that our lifestyle choices affect our health in profound ways. The field of wellness began with looking at health-risk behavior and tackled the challenge of helping our society reduce its health risks. Smoking cessation and weight control were at the forefront of this early effort with many of the fear-based programs intending to scare people into quitting smoking and reducing their weight. The emphasis was on reducing health risk factors and thereby reducing health related problems. Out of the movement came the health risk appraisals or assessments (HRAs) created to formally measure a person's health risk.

Over the years, more health correlations were made and we began to look at stress reduction, healthier interpersonal relationships, career satisfaction and other aspects of a person's life in order to get a complete picture of their health and well-being. Various models of wellness emerged and the value of concepts like "meaning and purpose" in life became recognized as central. The personal growth movement of the late sixties and early seventies spurred on the wellness movement and validated its base in the concept of personal growth, development and self-actualization.

In 1975, a physician who wanted to do more than just treat illness established the first wellness resource center (not a clinic). Jack Travis, developed a Marin County, California center to work with individuals who truly wanted to be well. Offering programs that helped people learn skills for well-being, it went light years beyond what we learned in health class. In addition to some of the expected how to be well information on better ways to exercise and eat, the Wellness

Resource Center emphasized the psychological as well. The Center placed emphasis on identifying and removing emotional barriers to being well, improving communication skills, enhancing creativity and learning deep relaxation techniques. And, in very coach-like fashion, it asked clients (not patients) to look at envisioning desired outcomes and taking full responsibility for their own health and wellbeing.

Travis' center worked with individuals to help them learn how to take charge of their own lives. The Center's clients worked with the early version of The Wellness Inventory (developed by Travis), as well as a Health Risk Appraisal and then created a plan for how to really live well. After the evaluation stage, clients enrolled in individual sessions with counselors and joined a lifestyle evolution group to help them learn the basics of wellness.

The Wellness Resource Center did not last many years though, and the center model did not catch fire. Companies looked to insurance and managed care as the answers. With the costs of health care beginning to rise, corporations began to look seriously upstream. Companies such as Progressive Insurance, Campbell Soup, Bayer, IBM, Coors, and others, looked to the growing field of health education and health promotion for wellness help.

Psychologist Robert Allen pioneered examining how health norms of the people we live and work with affect our health. In the workplace, programs were developed to influence the culture of the work environment. Many companies invested in physical fitness facilities for employees. Health-risk assessments were used on a broad scale. The emphasis was moved to health education and affecting large groups of people through classes, incentive programs, and various wellness health promotion efforts.

This was a step in the right direction and yet today health educators have found that in addition to the educative-classes-and-promotion approach, they are increasingly expected to work with individuals. Sometimes they have the skills to do so, other times they apply the training they know and attempt to simply educate the individual, hoping it will result in behavioral change. It often does not. Wellness is also becoming more consumer-driven. There is an increasing demand by individuals, outside of the workplace, for alliances that can help them, once and for all, be successful in changing their lifestyle behavior.

Many in the wellness field feel they been successful in some ways, and unsuccessful in others. Our culture-wide, society-wide or company-wide health promotion efforts have not been able to adequately improve the health of our country. There is encouragement instead of discouragement when we take wellness one-on-one. The new trend in wellness is helping improve the health of our world, one person at a time. It seems we are best served to come full circle to an individualized approach to wellness.

There is a tag-line joke that tells us "Chocolate! It's not just for breakfast anymore." We could say the same thing today about wellness and prevention. Indeed, much of the work in wellness, and especially wellness coaching, is more about lifestyle improvement as a way to positively affect the course of an illness. The new field of Lifestyle Medicine has grown at an astonishing rate as it embraces the evidence that shows us just how behavioral health really is.

*"Recent clinical research provides a strong evidential basis for the preferential use of lifestyle interventions as first-line therapy. This research is moving lifestyle from **prevention** only to include **treatment**--from an intervention used to **prevent disease** to an intervention used to **treat disease.**"*

The American College of Lifestyle Medicine (ACLM)

The ACLM goes on to say that "Lifestyle medicine is becoming the preferred modality for not only the prevention but the treatment of most chronic diseases, including: type-2 diabetes; coronary heart disease; hypertension; obesity; insulin resistance syndrome; osteoporosis; and many types of cancer." (www.lifestylemedicine.org).

Our view of wellness has been expanded ten-fold since the early days of the movement. Now, when we look at what wellness is and who is involved in it we must include not just health educators and health promotion experts, but thousands of enlightened healthcare professionals who see this merger of health and wellness. This interdisciplinary effort is breaking down the silos of health, medicine, behavioral health and wellness and helping us realize that we are all working on the same farm.

Individualizing Wellness:
The Coach Approach to Lifestyle Change

The wellness field has grown and been around for approximately thirty years. Changing the health behavior of the world has been a challenge, to say the least. In the United States, Canada, Europe, Australia, some parts of Asia and South America, the health efforts have been vigorous. In other areas the primary factor in overall health is not lifestyle, but living conditions, and there, wellness faces more unique challenges.

Throughout the thirty-year effort we discovered many approaches that worked and some that did not. Central to it all is a change in basic mindset that the approach to individual wellness has been based on.

Prescribe and Treat

As I began training wellness coaches and teaching coaching skills to wellness professionals, my students often reported that behavior change was so puzzling to them. "I tell them what to do, and they don't do it!" was often the exasperated cry.

Much of wellness is steeped in the great medical tradition. At times wellness professionals are working in medical clinics. Many times they are themselves nurses, therapists, or others trained in the medical model. That mindset is prescribe and treat, or diagnose, prescribe and treat. It is a mindset that was designed for remedial care. It is a mindset that works well in medical cases, and especially well when there is no behavioral compliance required by the patient.

In recent years we have seen the medical field extremely frustrated by the lack of patient compliance even with pharmaceutical prescriptions, much less behavioral directions from the doctor to alter one's lifestyle. Half the battle, they will tell you, in treating a newly diagnosed diabetic, is getting them to comply with directions for their own self-testing, diet, exercise and self-administration of treatment.

Unless there is no behavioral component to the treatment that requires the patient to follow-through in any way, the prescribe and treat method can be replete with difficulty. Just telling people what to do doesn't work well. The inherent authority of medical personnel just doesn't carry the same weight it used to. Although there may be acquiescence in the medical office, things may be quite different when the patient is on his/her own. Culture, lack of money, time limitations, access to conflicting information on the internet, all play a role that is not addressed in the current prescribe and treat system. When wellness work is carried out with this same prescriptive and admonishing approach we see results only when the client is truly ready and open to making the changes prescribed.

A 2012 meta-analysis published in the *Annals of Internal Medicine*, tells us that pharmaceutical noncompliance alone is totaling anywhere between $100 billion to $289 billion a year in healthcare costs in the Unites States. Filling a pharmaceutical prescription and then remembering and taking the medicine prescribed properly are all behavioral acts. Add to this the lifestyle prescriptions to change one's diet, exercise more and manage stress better, and we see that the issue of patient/client compliance is truly a critical behavioral health issue.

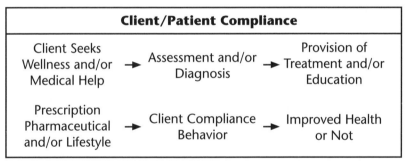

FIGURE 3.1

Whether applied to a treatment situation or to a wellness/health education situation, the final goal of improved health and wellbeing will only be reached if the flow is completed and there is client compliance. Success hinges on this crucial stage; if the client does not complete the process, all the previous efforts are to no avail.

There are treatment situations where the treatment provided immediately is sufficient. Administration of an appropriate medication may do the job, if the job is small enough. However, there is usually some kind of procedure that the patient needs to follow. That is where compliance comes in. So, as physiological as medicine is, its success is often determined by the psychological aspects. In the field of behavioral medicine we have come to say that there is nothing physiological, only psycho-physiological. We have come to realize that there is no separation between a person's mind and body. They work together and impact each other.

The other contradiction is that a prescribe and treat approach to wellness assumes that there is something wrong with the person. This seems to make the assumption that the wellness professional knows more about the client's body than the person consulting with them. The "I'm going to figure out what's wrong with you and tell you what to do about it" approach does not engage the person in his or her own wellness process.

Many wellness professionals are simply doing what they have been taught. Some students from the medical field have told me how they have been taught ways to cut off the input of the patient in order to save time and get to the diagnosis and prescription more quickly. Time is limited and emotional connection is discouraged. Wellness coaching is not medical interviewing.

Educate and Implore

Wellness professionals don't always take a medical approach. Some are trained as health educators. Being educators, they want to educate! The vast majority of wellness and health promotion is done in the belief that providing people with the best possible health information will result in improved health.

Certainly the importance of good, accurate health information cannot be criticized. We have seen great strides in public health since we begin teaching people to wash their hands (especially surgeons!) and not to sneeze on one another. We take it for granted today, but these simple maxims were not common practice only a hundred years ago. Establishing the link between smoking and a whole list of deadly diseases and getting the word out about it is just one example of heroic public health education. Now smoking is banned in public places in many states and countries.

There are those rare occasions when just the right information hits at just the right time. I experienced this when I read an alarming article on feedlot-raised beef. That was over 25 years ago and I haven't eaten beef since. However, when it comes to lifestyle behavioral change, information alone is insufficient most of the time.

All too often the health educator provides great information and delivers it in friendly, caring and often creative, ways to the person. Yet, there is often no change in behavior. They implore the person to use this great information and change. Still, there may be no change in behavior.

Health and wellness professionals are trained to conduct classes and do health promotion. Weight-loss classes are often just that—classes. The educator educates and there is hope that the students will take the information presented and transform their lives.

When the educative approach is attempted in a one-on-one situation, educate and implore just isn't enough. I would say that every one of the health educators I have worked with have been sincere about their job and have given it their very best effort. In fact, they often tell me that before they discovered the coach-approach, they thought that the more they talked (and provided great information) the better job they were doing. They truly wanted to give as much as possible to their client. Yet in retrospect, they realized how they often had overwhelmed their clients with information and left them in dazed confusion. Often there was no implementation of any of the great information that had been provided.

> *To hold and fill to overflowing*
> *is not as good as to stop in time.*
> *Sharpen a sword-edge to its very sharpest,*
> *And the edge will not last long.*
> *Withdraw as soon as your work is done.*
> *Such is Heaven's Way.*
>
> **–Lao Tzu**

Advocate and Inspire

With the recognition that so much of health and wellbeing is behavioral, we are at long last, acknowledging the need for a third professional to enter the scene. Joining the valued treatment providers and the health educators is the wellness coach. Taking a different stance than even the counselor or psychologist, who are still in the realm of treatment, the wellness coach is there to be an advocate for the client's health and wellbeing, to inspire and support their growth and development.

Operating with a mindset that is fundamentally different, the wellness coach is there to stand by the client, to stand with them, and stand next to them as a guide. Living in Colorado for many years, and exploring mountains around the world, I enjoy using the metaphor of the coach being like a mountain guide.

Mountain guides do not climb mountains for people. Nothing is accomplished, really, if you hire me as your mountain guide and pay me merely to plant your flag on the summit while you sip martinis and observe me through a telescope down at the lodge.

As your guide, I help you plan the climb. We assess your readiness for the climb, examine what you have and what you need in equipment and resources. Together we determine a route to take. We plan how long the journey will take and allow for elements we can't control, be it the weather or a family crisis. We examine what your personal goals are. Are you a peak-bagger, or more into the sheer experience of the high country? We get clear on what a successful and fulfilling climb will be for you.

Mountain guides do not make people climb mountains. The motivation for the climb has to be within the climber. During times of discouragement I may lend support, or even challenge you to reach a little deeper for strength I know you have. I also know that your chances of success are far greater if your motivation is internal. You WANT to climb this mountain! You are excited about it, and you anticipate that the journey will in itself be a large part of the pleasure of the experience. It works best when it is not fear-based motivation. You are not climbing the mountain because you are afraid what will happen if you don't!

Most importantly, your chances of success are far greater just because you aren't doing it alone. Knowing that I am there with you on the journey shifts your entire mental approach. You push through the temptation to turn back prematurely (as you may have done so often in the past) as you look over at me climbing beside you. You know

I will hold you accountable to yourself to do what you said you have come to do. You also know that you retain your freedom, and if you choose to turn back you will not be criticized for it. When we do summit, it is your flag that is planted, not mine, for this was your journey. It was you and the mountain. Your coach was like a good solid rope—a support.

The Mindset Shift—Being an Ally

The wellness professional sees everything new as if through a different lens once they make the mindset shift to that of an ally. Doing so may not be easy. In addition to the sheer power of habit, there may be some attraction remaining to the older models. Look inside and ask if you are ready to become an ally to your patient/client instead of a teacher or medical authority. Some people have higher needs for control than others. Being a wellness ally requires letting go of those needs for control and distance.

Another part of the mindset shift is a shift in responsibility. As an ally you work with a person to make their own changes. They, not you, are ultimately responsible for changing their own behavior. In fact, part of the coach approach is supporting the client's acceptance of more and more responsibility for their own health and their own life. To do anything else encourages a co-dependency that works against the client, not for them.

Shifting the emphasis from education and provision of services to the role of an ally is indeed a different role. The services we provide are actions done with the client, not to them or for them. At first it may seem that we aren't doing enough for the client, but as we see them grow and change, we realize that our alliance is making a truly significant difference.

Four Cornerstones of Coaching

One of the most beautiful alignments of wellness and coaching is in the "cornerstones of coaching" set forth in the book *Co-Active Coaching* by coach education pioneers Laura Whitworth, Henry Kimsey-House and Phil Sandahl.

Cornerstone One: Clients are naturally creative, resourceful and whole. The wellness approach and the coaching approach both see the client as OK the way they are, nothing to be fixed, nothing to be treated. The client is whole and complete, just they way they are, and the coach accepts them as such. That is not to say that real health challenges are ignored. However, the person with the health challenge is seen as OK, as a resourceful, creative and complete human being who wants to grow. The leg may be broken, but the person is not!

This mindset shift becomes operational in many ways. When you adopt the mindset of the wellness ally your interaction with your client or patient changes on a number of levels.

- Intention shifts. We are all masters of perceiving, largely through non-verbal communication, and perhaps on other perceptual levels harder to study, the intention of people we are communicating with. What is the intention of the healthcare provider who is providing treatment? Hopefully to heal, but even that can come across as fixing, as a judgment that there is something wrong with the patient that needs fixing. This is the most common doctor-patient agreement—just give me a pill and send me home. However, the patient is now asking to be part of healing process and is not seeking to be fixed. So there needs to be a new intention. Now the client is looking for an ally who respects his/her own ability to help him/herself, and needs what that alliance can provide to ensure success.

- Closeness shifts. When we meet a client as an ally we sit beside them, not above them, and we work at the development of trust. We are open to more closeness than before. We demonstrate this openness to our client and present an invitation to trust and to deepen our experience of each other in our professional relationship. Many a student of medicine, nursing and therapy got the advice I received my sophomore year as a psychology major from a veteran professor and clinician. "Don't get too close to your patients!" There are some legitimate reasons for therapeutic distance. Clinical judgment can be impaired by personal feelings. Burnout prevention may require the art of compassionate detachment. The beauty of this different coaching position is that we are not sitting in clinical judgment we are free to be a professional ally.

- Clients have the answers: Another way the coaching field acknowledges the nature of this alliance is with the pearl of wisdom that "The client has the answers, the coach has the questions." We are engaged in a process to help clients find their own answers that they really do have within themselves. We don't motivate anyone! We help them find (gain access to) the motivation they have within themselves.

To work from this perspective requires us, as the wellness ally, to let go of the expert role. As a consultant it can feel very good to provide the kind of information a client finds helpful. At times, the coach can do this. We can direct a client to a resource that may help them or even make a specific suggestion. In the coach approach, though, we always ask the client for their permission, and we check out their desire. "Would you like to hear a suggestion I have about that?" We then offer our suggestion for the client to decide to accept or reject. Contrast that with the professional who is working in the role of expert and telling a person directly what they should do.

To let go of the expert role may require some work on our own self-confidence. It is easy to over-work, over-provide and over-educate (all called over-talking!) when inside we doubt ourselves. Clinging to that white uniform and the expert role we distance and protect ourselves, staying on what we might call the helpful offensive when working with a client.

To be present, to be dancing in the moment as we like to call it in coaching, we are required to be more centered about who we are and comfortable with just that. Many times as a coach I urge them to ask themselves "Who do I need to be?" instead of "What do I need to do?" The same is true for the wellness ally. Who do you need to be? What aspects of your character needs to show up, to be present, as you work with your client to serve them best in a coach-like way?

Cornerstone Two: Coaching addresses the client's whole life. In my first group teleconference call that introduced me further to the field of coaching, our host was drawing upon his extensive CEO business background for examples. Speaking for myself and several other therapists on the call, I asked what did we non-business background people have to bring to coaching. He laughed and said "You know, I'll tell you all something. All, yes, all of the business coaching I've done, at some point became life coaching." He went on to tell us—and I learned over the years that it was absolutely true—it wasn't lack of information that kept the business person from being more successful, it was their own personal characteristics, self-defeating behaviors, limiting self-beliefs and interpersonal skills (or the lack thereof) that determined their success. In wellness coaching, the same principle is true.

Tug on anything at all and you'll find it connected to
everything else in the universe.
—John Muir

When we really look at health and wellness, the atomistic, bio-medical model only takes us so far. The great rise of integrative health-care can largely attribute its powerful emergence to the fact that it focuses on the whole person. When we look at lifestyle improvement we quickly realize that it is a holistic concept. The sedentary, overweight client doesn't need just another prescription for a 1500 calorie diet, they need to look at how they are living their life, how they feel about themselves, where the support in their life comes from, and much more. They are not a person in isolation. They are part of other systems we know as family, workplace and community.

In wellness coaching we help our clients assess their wellness by looking at all aspects of their lives, three hundred and sixty degrees. A narrow behavioral approach to changing individual behaviors proves to be quite myopic when it comes to helping people with real lifestyle change. We identify areas for exploration, and sometimes it is surprising where the real benefits come from and where the keys to change are found.

Cornerstone Three: The agenda comes from the client. The coaching model thoroughly embraces the idea of operating in what is basically a client-centered way. Like the counseling approach developed by Carl Rogers, we stay with the client and go where they lead. As we apply this to wellness coaching we see that it is, again, a mindset shift from the medical or treatment model. It is even different than an approach a business consultant might take (the consultant knows best).

It may be very apparent to the wellness professional that the person they are talking with needs to quit smoking, exercise more, manage their stress better or find more supportive relationships. When the wellness professional takes this assessment and shoves it at the client as a recommendation it is very easy for it to be perceived as a prescription, or worse, as a judgment. This person doesn't feel like an ally. Clients are often resistant to such an approach and most often will comply while in the conversation and then not follow through, or will even drop out of participation.

The wellness coach may ask "What do you want to do? What are you ready to do?" In the coach approach we trust in the wisdom of the client and support them in what they are ready to work on. Nothing succeeds like success. Once the client experiences success in the first wellness goal they work on, they are more ready, willing and able to tackle another goal that they may gain even more benefit from.

> *Always remember that you are absolutely unique.*
> *Just like everyone else.*
>
> **–Margaret Mead**

Clients have friends and family who want to help, but they all have their own agenda. Family members may want the best for the client, but they would like it to look a certain way.

- Don't rock the boat.

- Don't be too assertive, we like having you do everything for us!

- Go out more, but not with him or her!

- Take time to have fun, but not too much time because we really need you to make more money.

- Take care of yourself, but oh, please don't cut down on the overtime you are doing for us.

One of the most refreshing things about coaching is that clients get to talk about their lives with someone who doesn't have to live with them or work with them, or even be related to them! Yes! The only agenda is the client's agenda!

When a wellness coach co-creates a wellness plan with a client, it is just that, co-creation. A plan is crafted together from the agenda the client sets. That's not to say the coach might not challenge the client to go for more, or coach them to attempt less. Like an athletic coach who believes in the ability of a player to perform better, the wellness coach might challenge the client to stretch themselves a bit. The coach may, on the other hand, see that more is being bitten off than is likely to be chewed and rather than creating a setup for failure may suggest taking on less. When all is said and done, the client remains behind the wheel—steering their life toward higher levels of wellness.

Cornerstone Four: The relationship is a designed alliance. Very consciously the coach and the client fashion a professional relationship that is a custom fit, instead of a one-size-fits-all treatment or education program. The goal is to create a relationship that matches the role of the coach with the kind of coaching the client needs. In the very first session, once it is clear that coaching is what the client wants, the first work of the new alliance is to create itself, and to do so in a conscious and unique way.

I often start a discovery session (the first session with a new client) by asking "What is the best way for me to coach you?" Often clients are not shy about telling me! Sometimes they really need an explanation of what the choices are and all the different ways that coaching can look. We all need accountability, but how much and in what manner? Are you a client who works best with a light rein or with really firm deadlines?

Agreements are created, not only about the more interpersonal aspects of working together, but the concrete and practical as well. Coaching agreements spell out fees, policies, etc. in real detail so everyone is clear.

With this new mindset and reliance on these cornerstones you are being more coach-like, and have a new way to interact with your clients. When you give your client an ally instead of an expert, and then stand with them, and stand by them through the change process, the client feels the support needed to succeed.

> *A safe and courageous space for change must be, by definition, a place where the truth can be told. It is a place where clients can tell the whole truth about what they have done (and not done) without worrying about looking good. This is an environment without judgment. And it is a place where the coach expects the truth from the client because there is no consequence of truth other than growth and learning.*
>
> **—L. Whitworth, H. Kimsey-House, P. Sandahl**
> *Co-Active Coaching*

The New Four Cornerstones of Coaching

In 2011, Henry, Karen and Philip (without Laura, whom the coaching world lost in 2007) put out a new third edition of their landmark book *Co-Active Coaching*. In it was a new version of The Four Cornerstones of Coaching.

1. People Are Naturally Creative Resourceful and Whole.
2. Focus on the Whole Person
3. Dance in This Moment
4. Evoke Transformation

The first two are essentially the same as has been written about here, but I want to add that as the authors speak of the first Cornerstone, they clarify something important. They state that when they say that people are naturally creative, resourceful and whole, they aren't just putting forth a model or a theory, they are taking a stand! I've often heard the first Cornerstone stated almost like a pledge by coaches "We hold our clients to be – naturally creative, resourceful and whole." It is seen as an assertion of something that is fundamentally true, something absolutely wired into all human beings.

At the Real Balance Wellness Coach Training Institute one of our faculty members told me that when she was learning to be a coach, she wrote NCRW in ink on the palm of her hand when she went into a coaching session so that she would constantly remember to maintain that honoring coaching mindset as she coached.

Let's take a look at the two newer Cornerstones.

Dance In This Moment

When great coaches speak of "dancing in the moment" they usually do so with a satisfied smile on their faces. One of the real joys in coaching is getting to the point where you aren't awkwardly trying to remember "left foot, left foot, right…" instead you are able to improvise, to flow with your dance partner. It's not like a prescribed-step dance, it's much freer than that. What determines the "moves" is the moment. What is happening in this very moment?

Was it the way your client's voice got soft and trailed off as they "agreed" to a new action step that they would take to help lose weight this week? Perhaps that tone said "I'm not so sure of this!" The coach who is a good dancer hears that tone of voice and instead of neatly finishing up the session with a new piece of accountability about the new action step, stops and checks things out with their client. How okay are they with this new commitment? Do they see the value in it? The coach might feedback their observation of that shift in tone and explore. The music might not be over yet!

Dancing in the moment means being willing to go with your client, sometimes following them, sometimes taking the lead by giving feedback, sharing observations, asking a challenging question, or asking permission to make a suggestion. It's like being one of those dancers you see on the floor who truly follows the beat of the music, adjusting along the way, instead of just moving with the same rhythm like they do to every song. Agility is a hallmark of a great coach.

Evoke Transformation

Coaching is so much about change. A change in behavior, in performance, in accomplishment, in attitude and belief. Yet, it is about so much more. Again, the founders of the coaching movement and the wellness movement have always been on the same page. Wellness, real wellness, is about personal growth and maximizing human potential. Excellent coaching is about assisting people in creating and living their best life possible.

As we co-create a Wellness Plan with our clients we often drill down to the specific action steps the client sees value in working on for this week. Yet, for maximum motivation there needs to be a link all the way back to their Well-Life Vision. They have to see the point in walking four times this week. The specific relates to the bigger picture. Sometimes our clients make the most progress when they have a coach who sees the true potential, the real capacity that their client has, even when the client cannot yet see it themselves. When our clients catch up with a sense of their own potential and see how their actions in the coaching progress are helping them maximize it, that is true transformation, not just "change".

> *"There is a yearning for the very best, the full potential that the coachee can experience. And when that connection ignites between today's goal and life's potential, the effect is transformative."*
>
> ***Co-Active Coaching* – Third Edition**

Chapter 4

Seven Steps to Lasting Lifestyle Change: Lifestyle Improvement Model

What is the most rigorous law of our being? Growth.
No smallest atom of our moral, mental, or physical structure
can stand still a year. It grows—it must grow;
nothing can prevent it.

—Mark Twain

There are many wonderful books available which tell us how to be well. They are great resources and more information is always valuable. What I am striving to do in this book, however, is to provide more in the way of exploring how we change our lifestyle. This involves behavior change. This is a territory worth exploring because it seems to be grounded where the trails are faint and elusive. Many a journey into this realm comes to a halt and the person turns around, retraces their steps and goes back where they came from. What blocks us from really getting far enough down that trail towards wellness to realize success? How do we block ourselves? What keeps us stuck at the trailhead, maintaining a lifestyle that at the minimum is keeping us from realizing our fullest potential, or, at it's worst, is killing us? What intrigues us about exploring this trail leading off over some hill and into the unknown? What motivates us to start the journey of a thousand miles with our first step? These are questions that have always fascinated me.

Present Lifestyle

We always begin the journey where we are, in the present. We review our present lifestyle to see what it looks like and how it is being maintained. Our current lifestyle is always maintained by some combination of habit, comfort, fear and reinforcement. While one could argue that there are many ways that these elements overlap and combine, let's look at each separately.

Many of the habits with which we live our lives are efficient ways of behaving, serving us well and saving us time and energy. I brush my teeth pretty much the same way, the same times of day, without a whole lot of thought. My dental hygienist might show me a better way of brushing my teeth, but chances are good that I will just continue in my old habitual way unless I engage is some kind of real change process. Other habits may be quite neutral or may have a severe negative impact on our level of wellness. At the very least, one of the most insidious aspects of habit is that it dulls our awareness. When I drive to work the same way everyday I may notice less about the world around me than when I vary the route. Noticing less about the world around us contributes less to our growth and the enjoyment of our experience. Noticing less may mean a traffic wreck. Today it is the driver running the stoplight in front of us and in ancient times it was the growl of the saber-tooth tiger. Awareness is one of the keys to our survival, and also one of the keys to our living a delightful life! When I am more aware I notice the beauty of the world as well as the dangers. I notice the flowers beside the sidewalk as well as the crack that may trip me.

Habits can be so ingrained that even when we identify them for change, the process is not easy. Most people have a pretty good idea of some important changes they would like to make in their lifestyle. The power of habit often keeps them stuck. They make up their minds to change a behavior and then criticize themselves harshly when sheer will power isn't enough to overcome a long-standing and deeply rooted habit. We'll explore how to work through and change a habit later in this book.

"I'm into creature comforts!" a friend of mine used to say. His idea of a great lifestyle was richly marbled steaks, good aged scotch, a plush lounge chair and satellite television. As you might expect, since this was his way of living on a regular basis, not just an occasional enjoyment, he was overweight, in very poor physical condition, and while he certainly knew how to relax, his health was walking a very thin line. This fellow was an extreme case, but we all know how many of our lifestyle choices are swayed by what simply gives us the most comfort. The lure of the couch can be powerful, as can the comfort that comes from foods that remind us of home, warmth and relaxation. While there is nothing wrong with comfort—in fact some people need to seek much more of it in their self-denying lives—balance is really the goal. Unfortunately, the habitual need for comfort can keep us stuck in very unhealthy lifestyles.

Change creates loss. Even if the change is positive, we have to let go of something. Fear of change is fear of loss and fear that we may not be able to adapt to the changing environment. There seems to be a little voice inside all of us that shouts "Status quo!" and fights change with tooth and nail. The more a person lives in fear the smaller they make their world. People reduce their options and choices in order to stay safe. They pass judgments on others to eliminate having to deal with them and perhaps encounter the forces of change. We fear failure and we fear success.

For many people lifestyle improvement is an area where they have already experienced the pain of many failures. Usually alone, they have tried to quit smoking, lose weight, be more intimate in close relationships, etc., and their efforts have only seemed to cause pain. Why try again? Discouragement feeds the fear and unfortunately there is much in the world around us that reinforces a very unhealthy lifestyle. Our peer group or family may exhibit unhealthy habits and find connection with us through these habits. It's hard to be the only person in a work group who brings their own bag lunch when everyone else takes a break together at the fast-food restaurant. It's tough for the college student to have just a couple of beers at the binge-drinking party. Why get out and hike or bike on the weekend when everyone else in the family is into movies, video games and television?

Beyond peer norms, however, is the phenomenal impact of a culture where gigantic profits are made from the promotion of unhealthy living. Mass media constantly challenges our efforts at a healthy lifestyle with billions of dollars of advertising promoting industrialized food, gas-guzzling pollution-mobiles, sugar-loaded beverages, and the message that materialism is the way to true happiness. A quick review of Eric Schlosser's book *Fast Food Nation*, or Morgan Spurlock's film *Super-size Me* will raise awareness of how the simple goal of greater profitability has cast human health aside.

The bottom line is that these forces in our society do have an impact on us, even though we all certainly have the ability to make our own choices. Free will may be a reality, but all that we have learned from social psychology would argue that it's not that simple.

The Desire to Change

When a wellness professional sees all the factors at work to hold a person's present lifestyle in stagnation, how can they hope to assist people to change? One of the continually remarkable and fascinating things about human beings is our desire to set out for the great unknown. Despite a dozen reasons to stay where we are, time and time again, we search for a better life and make our attempts at growth and change. What moves or motivates this desire for change? Love and fear are primary motivators. We are either moving towards something or away from something.

Psychiatrist Gerry Jampolsky (*Love Is Letting Go of Fear*) has long shared the wisdom from *A Course In Miracles*, that everything we do comes either from love or from fear. When we apply this to the lifestyle change arena we see that fear is motivating us not into fight or flight but into freeze or flight. Just like a rabbit in the brush as the hunter comes near, we might find that our fear causes us to become immobilized. We may fear the diagnosis, so we never go in for the exam! However, when we flush into flight, it is fear motivating us to take action. As Bill Cosby said in a comedy routine about the grim subject of cancer, "I figure if I don't go in and get the exam then the doctor can't tell me I've got it, and if he doesn't tell me that I've got it...then I ain't got it!"

A good wellness assessment tool may alert us to risks that are shortening the chances for us to have a long and healthy life. A new diagnosis or health incident may alarm us and motivate change. We may act out of fear of death or a life of disability. At the same time our motivation for change may come out of love of self.

It may be the love that we have for ourselves that motivates our desire to maintain life and health. It may be the love that we have for others who love and care about us. Many people quit smoking either to help their children avoid second-hand smoke, or out of a pledge they make to themselves to be around longer for those children or grandchildren.

Fear is often a great springboard for change. It can jolt us into taking action. Sustaining that action, however, is where fear begins to lose its effectiveness. One of the primary reasons for having a wellness coach is to succeed in lifestyle change where the client may have failed (perhaps repeatedly) in the past. When we look for change that lasts, when we look for the motivation to carry the person through the replacement of negative health habits with positive ones, we need to look to love. We will cover the motivational aspects of how to do this later in this book, but clearly self-esteem, self-love, is a well to be tapped to sustain our desire for change. Tapping into the innate self-loving forces that strive for self-actualization accesses a powerful energy that fuels change.

Seven Steps for Lasting Lifestyle Improvement

The pursuit of higher levels of wellness can take many forms. When we look at ways that wellness professionals and wellness coaches can help people in this process, this is one model to consider.

Seven Steps for Lasting Lifestyle Improvement

1. Assessment

In any change process it is important for a person to assess where they are and what they want to accomplish. Self-assessment, feedback from others, and evaluation tools all can help determine the current level of functioning in different areas or life dimensions. Looking at the whole person, the coach helps the client determine their readiness to change specific behaviors and assists him/her to set a direction.

We all need to develop the ability to observe ourselves. Taking stock of our wellness through some kind of thorough review process increases our self awareness and helps us determine areas to focus on. Again, some of the irony in wellness is that, for such a holistic concept, where we realize that every aspect of our lives is inextricably linked to every other aspect, we need to break it down into pieces we can work with. Mind, body, spirit and environment all benefit from examination.

As a coach you ask your clients questions with a specific purpose. Rather than gathering data for a diagnosis, you are instead posing questions that help your clients dig down and gain insights into how and why they do things. In your initial work with clients much can be gained by a supportive and patient exploration, in conversational form, of clients' current life and lifestyle. Avoid why questions and explore the what and the how of the client's life. Help them to put descriptions of their experiences into words. In doing so, your clients are required to observe, review, synthesize, and communicate about their experience in a way that is very different from just thinking about it to themselves. Realizations may emerge for your clients during this time and you can help to capture and work them into an effective wellness plan.

Part of self-assessment is getting current information on one's health status. An up-to-date and thorough medical examination may yield critical information. The healthcare team may have important recommendations for ways your client needs to improve their life-style. Coach and client can then integrate this s "lifestyle prescription" into the wellness plan.

Wellness assessment tools provide valuable feedback for clients and often get at areas that might otherwise be ignored. Health risk assessments (HRA's), instruments like The Wellness Inventory, and Test Well, help the client expand their awareness of how they are functioning in the life dimension areas included in the specific instrument.

As the work of James Prochaska, et. al. in *Changing For Good* reminds us, people don't change until they are ready to. A key part of the assessment phase of this model is helping your clients to realize which stage of change they are in with regard to each behavior they would like to improve, and how they currently define improvement.

2. Foundational Work On Self

Before any goal setting can be truly effective, action must be taken to increase awareness of self on environmental, interpersonal, intraper-sonal, and spiritual levels. Exploration of various wellness teachings and systems are beneficial and may be carried out during this step.

It is tempting to simplify wellness work into a system of identifying something to work on, setting a goal and following up on progress. Sometimes this is adequate. When we look at how often lifestyle change efforts fail, perhaps we need to help the client dig a little deeper.

The original concept of wellness was rooted in the model of personal growth. When we help clients become excited about their own personal growth process the motivation for wellness becomes much more intrinsic. Supporting clients in their journey of self-exploration, and giving them permission and encouragement to do so helps access this internal drive to actualize potential and engage in change.

As a wellness coach you may find that some of your clients are not terribly introspective. This is not always some kind of defensiveness or resistance, it may just be who they are. If they are great at co-creating a wellness plan with you and then vigilant at self-monitoring (tracking their behavior) there may not be any need for great personal insights. However, if there are internal and external barriers in the way that have arisen before blocking progress, then a deeper look may pay off.

Foundational work on one's self requires a good, hard look at one's life, not just one's lifestyle. Values may need to be clarified. Time set aside for introspection and reflection may yield a more accurate vision of the changes that are really important for this person at this time in their life.

3. Setting the Focus

Desired outcomes become clear from the foundational work done in areas that a client wants to focus on. Wellness action steps are developed that are designed to move clients toward the desired outcomes in these areas of focus.

Combining the information from the assessment phase with the realizations and insights of the foundational work on self, the coach helps clients to determine what they are ready, willing, and able to work on now and in the near future. A wellness plan is co-created. All the exploration and steps are brought together into this wellness plan.

Conscious awareness is what distinguishes a wellness lifestyle. It is with conscious awareness and thoughtfulness that a step-by-step plan is forged. Together the client and coach ask "Where do we want to go? How will we know when we've arrived?"

The wellness plan is an agreement for action. As the wellness plan is put into effect, agreements are formed about accountability. One of the real strengths of the coach approach is the way in which it helps a client hold themselves accountable to themselves. No more empty self-promises. Effective wellness coaching accountability is escape-proof.

4. Working Through Habit + Environmental Support

Old habits are overcome through repeated, patient and persistent action. When no longer desired habits re-emerge they are accepted as evidence of their truly habitual nature and discouragement is avoided. During this phase a person needs to develop a supportive environment for lifestyle change to occur. We need peer health norms that support healthy changes, such as alliances with friends and wellness professionals support consistent action for healthy change.

As your wellness coaching client begins the actual process of behavioral change they are soon confronted with the power of habit. Lifestyles are defined by habit. The less awareness a person has, the greater the habitual power of the behavior will have over them. Most clients vow to change a certain behavior and when it re-emerges they blame themselves and make it a matter of lacking will power or strength of character. The wellness coach can truly serve their client well by reminding them of the true nature of habitual behavior and encouraging them to accept this and celebrate their success in noticing and catching the old behavior.

We now know that habits are literally wired into our brains. Neuroscience is showing us that changing habits is not as simple as making a New Year's Resolution. Functional MRI research has shown us the brain in action and we've discovered that our strongest habits have formed greater neural pathways there. The neurons that fire together, wire together. So when our middle-aged client is attempting to change a daily habit, some combination of thinking and action that they have performed thousands of times over twenty or thirty years or more, its no wonder that they find it challenging. Its not just about "will-power" and the re-emergence of the old habit is not evidence of weak character.

Friends do keep friends healthy. By strategizing with you, the wellness coach, your client can consciously seek out more and more environmental support for their wellness efforts. We will look at how to "coach for connectedness" later in this book.

5. Initial Behavioral Change

When we see initial success it is accepted and celebrated and not minimized. Seen as *initial* success, it is also recognized that more work remains. As resistance patterns emerge they are noted and addressed but not focused on endlessly.

Many clients tend to discount or minimize their successes. Sometimes, without a wellness ally, they don't even recognize when they have made progress. Especially early in the behavioral change process, it is paramount to identify successes and to celebrate and reinforce them.

Experiencing initial change in a particular behavior is often something the client has experienced before, but which did not last. Alone, it is easy to see some progress and then to revert back to old patterns and discouragement, even abandonment of all efforts at the desired change. Here you can play a vital role by not only keeping your client on task through accountability and support, but by helping them become conscious of their experience of the process. This is the time to tweak the wellness plan. Resistance patterns need to be identified and examined and the goals may need to be re-evaluated and perhaps re-adjusted.

6. Deeper Work On Self

Higher levels of self-awareness, fear and resistances are explored in this phase. The spiritual elements and emotional issues become primary. Systems of exploration learned earlier are used as tools to find the answers to both internal and external barriers.

Experiencing change, even positive change, can bring up fear. Changes in lifestyle ripple through our lives affecting our relationships with others and engaging issues not previously thought about. A client who decides to drink less and less often must now deal with his or her drinking buddies who want to continue to party hard and often. A positive increase in setting boundaries and saying no to people can have totally unpredicted reactions by others. You may not be acting like the person people learned to care about or used to play with. Sometimes it brings up emotional closeness issues or trust and loss issues that may require reaching deeper inside to find the courage to maintain the changes.

As wellness coach you can also work with your client to explore this experience of "push-back" by the world around them. Strategic coaching can help your client come up with new ways of approaching others with improved communication, appropriate assertiveness, or whatever is most effective to move through these barriers to change.

Knee-deep in the change process, clients sometimes exhibit self-defeating behavior based on self-limiting beliefs about themselves and the world around them. The inner-critic absolutely abhors change and at this stage usually floods the client with all the lies they are willing to listen to about themselves. This has often been the place where discouragement takes over and previous wellness efforts were abandoned.

When this happens, the coach helps clients as they take their journey into the heart of self. If clients choose to explore old wounds and to do some deep healing, then a referral to psychotherapy is more in order than coaching. Coaching can go on simultaneously during therapy to continue progress on lifestyle improvement goals. The coach can continue to be an ally as the client searches for the answers that lie within.

7. Lasting Behavioral/Lifestyle Change

The lifestyle change has taken hold and the benefits of the change are the motivation. It has become part of the current lifestyle habits of the client. Periodic re-assessment maintains awareness and identifies new areas for attention. Alliances with friends and wellness professionals support the continuation of healthy lifestyle behavior. In this phase centering practices solidify and help maintain lifestyle improvements. Clients experience and enjoy good health and celebrate in joyous action.

Success is experienced and now the work is one of maintaining the successful change. As Prochaska points out in his Stages of Change model, until the new behaviors become almost automatic, the job is not done. Addiction models have taught us about relapse and there is a wellness equivalent. Now, the wellness coach helps reinforce the success and creates strategies with the client to maintain it. Self-efficacy feelings have to be high and alliances with others at home and work solid to assure that the changes will endure. Connectedness and social support now ensure lasting success. Agreements for periodic re-assessments will help keep the client vigilant and identify newly emerging areas to work on.

Personal growth has no end point. While coaching may be over, the client is encouraged to see their life as a continually evolving adventure.

> *The journey into self-love and self-acceptance must begin with self-examination . . . until you take the journey of self-reflection, it is almost impossible to grow or learn in life.*
>
> **—Iyanla Van Zant**, *Until Today*

Chapter 5

Becoming a Wellness Coach

So, faith is no more than the willingness and bravery to enter
and ride the stream. The mystery is that taking the risk to
be so immersed in our moment of living in itself joins us
with everything larger than us. And what is compassion but
entering the stream of another without losing yourself?

—**Mark Nepo,** *The Book of Awakening*

The helping professions attract wonderful people who are committed to serving others and making the world a better place. As interests and talents combine with what people believe about themselves and their own life circumstances, career directions develop. Some become social workers, some nurses, physicians, counselors, psychologists, and therapists of many varieties. A few even become wellness educators. For the most part though, wellness is not so much a profession as it is a way to practice one's profession.

The recently birthed profession of coaching sprang from the marriage of the business world and the world of psychology, counseling, etc. Coaching, and life coaching in particular, brought with it a set of competencies that are proving valuable throughout not only the business world, but the helping professions as well. When people graduate from reputable coach training schools, they gain expertise based on some of the most effective and cutting edge knowledge in the areas of communication, problem solving, creativity, conflict resolution and more.

Who Becomes a Wellness Coach

Wellness coaches seem to emerge from two primary sources; coaches who are drawn to wellness, and wellness professionals who are drawn to coaching. Life coaches discover that they can combine long-standing personal and professional interests in wellness and/or holistic health with the skills of their coaching training. Despite their own backgrounds in coaching and perhaps even in therapy, they may or may not be familiar with many of the concepts that have been developed by the wellness field and the related professions. The challenge is to learn what wellness truly is and the key concepts that form the basis of effective lifestyle behavioral change. Understanding wellness theories, assessments, and foundational concepts, such as readiness for change theory, are extremely helpful to the life coach.

For the wellness professional the challenge is learning one-on-one skills and how to apply them in their wellness work. While they may be very familiar with wellness and lifestyle improvement concepts and principles, their academic and on-the-job training is usually devoid of interpersonal skills work. If they did receive any client interview training, it may have been from the medical treatment model orientation of diagnostic data gathering. The skills of coaching open their eyes to a whole new world of interaction with their clients/patients.

Many wellness professionals decide to combine the mindset shift and skills of coaching with their existing wellness work. One example would be physical fitness trainers who add coaching to the fitness training work that they do. Such a person may or may not actually practice as a "wellness coach," but may simply be more "coach-like" in the way they do their work. This can be a very valuable shift for the wellness educator, the nurse practitioner, the diabetes educator, etc., as they interact with patients/clients in a more effective and productive way.

Some wellness professionals decide to complete training as a professional coach and either establish their own independent work, or function as a wellness coach within an existing organizational setting. Theirs is a more complete shift in professions and their work helping people make lasting lifestyle change now operates more completely from a coaching foundation.

. . . character transforms while persona copes.

—Kevin Cashman (*Leadership From The Inside Out*)

What Makes a Good Coach

Williams and Davis, in their book, *Therapist As Life Coach*, list 20 characteristics that people who are drawn to coaching tend to have. Which ones are strengths of yours? Which ones do you wish to develop more?

1. They are well adjusted and constantly seek personal improvement or development.
2. They have a lightness of being and *joi de vivre*.
3. They are passionate about "growing" as people.
4. They understand the distinction and balance between *being* and *doing*.
5. They are able to suspend judgment and stay open-minded.
6. They are risk-takers willing to get out of their own comfort zones.
7. They are entrepreneurial—even if they do not have great business skills they are visionaries, able to see the big picture and reinvent themselves and their business to meet current trends.
8. They want to have a life as well as a business.
9. They have a worldview and a more global vision.
10. They are naturally motivational and optimistic.
11. They are great listeners who are able to empathize with their clients.
12. They are mentally healthy and resilient when life knocks them down.
13. Their focus is on developing the future, not fixing the past.
14. They are able to collaborate and partner with their clients, shedding the "expert" role.
15. They have a willingness to believe in the brilliance or potential for greatness in all people.
16. They look at possibilities instead of problems and causes.
17. They exude confidence, even when unsure.
18. They present as authentic and genuine, with high integrity.
19. They are willing to say, "I don't know," and explore where and how to learn what is needed.
20. They enjoy what they do and are enthusiastic and passionate about life.

While wellness coaches may, or may not, have as many entrepreneurial and business-oriented tendencies, they do share these 20 characteristics, plus ten more:

1. They are committed to living the healthiest lifestyle possible.
2. They have fairly low needs for control.
3. They tend to be very centered emotionally and calm in a crisis.
4. They are patient, but not indulgent or enabling with their clients.
5. They tend to see patterns and be good systems thinkers.
6. They love to strategize and develop new ways to do things.
7. They believe that mind, body, spirit and environment all contribute to health and wellbeing.
8. They embrace challenges instead of fearing them.
9. They are perpetually curious about life in general and human behavior in particular.
10. They are life-long learners.

Getting Professional Training to Be a Coach

Learning to be more coach-like in the wellness work you do can be achieved best from direct training in coaching skills. The excitement about wellness coaching as a model for individualizing wellness services is driving some folks to just jump headlong into attempting one-on-one work after having just read a book and few articles. Winging it will only go so far, and the danger is that the newly self-proclaimed coach (or dubbed to be such by the organization) will not have the theoretical background, awareness of when to refer to treatment, and the actual powerful communication skills that are the foundation of coaching. These coaches may have more difficulty staying in the coach mindset and continue to revert back to the old models of prescribe and treat or educate and implore. Some wellness veterans who have been doing one-on-one work for years may benefit tremendously from discovering how the profession of coaching can hone their skills and give them an even more effective mindset and background.

Nothing beats live training with a qualified and experienced wellness coach/trainer and many trainers travel internationally. Fully interactive online webinair and teleconference courses in coaching are a close second. Many in the coaching profession feel that the highly interpersonal/interactive skills of coaching cannot and should not be attempted with solely online (computer based) learning. This is not a matter of studying data. It is learning both shifts in mindset and actual interactive skills that require practice, demonstration and feedback.

When a wellness professional wants to go in the direction of becoming qualified as a professional coach, seeking out training from recognized and certified schools is best. The first criterion would be looking for a coach training school that is certified by the International Coaching Federation (ICF). Meeting the rigorous standards of the ICF requires that a school offer quality courses taught by qualified and competent instructors. It is quality assurance that the student will receive the education they are promised and a certification that has respect. Equivalent certifications can be found offered in countries other than the United States. Though the ICF is indeed international, you may find other quality standard measures in your country.

With today's sophisticated world-wide communication systems, it is quite possible to receive coach training via webinair or teleconference calls from anywhere in the world. These may require some very early morning or late night calls from your time zone, however! You may also be able to enlist a mentor coach to provide individualized coach training.

Look for Wellness Coach Training

While some coaching schools offer a good life coach training program, not all may contain actual training in the specialty of wellness coach training. Missing from their programs may be emphasis on how to adapt coaching to the area of lifestyle behavioral change, and the theoretical and practical information from the wellness and health promotion fields that are essential to effective wellness coaching. Look for programs that offer you either complete training in wellness coaching or include a firm foundation in life coaching and also train specifically in wellness coaching as a specialty area.

Your Personal Wellness Foundation

Your credibility as a wellness coach depends to a great extent upon your dedication to your own wellness. This is truly an area where you must walk your talk. That doesn't mean you have already achieved physical, mental/emotional and spiritual perfection, or complete self-actualization. It means you are dedicated to working on improving your lifestyle, your health and wellbeing, and in the process of self-actualization. This will be quite evident and very inspiring to your clients.

There are a number of great rationales for continual work on your own Personal Wellness Foundation (PWF).

1. Doing so lends credibility and integrity to your work.
2. Your level of empathy and understanding is increased.
3. You will prevent burnout.
4. You continue to learn as both a provider and a consumer of wellness.

Your ability to appropriately self-disclose about your own wellness journey can be a real asset to the client's coaching experience. The worst coaching comes from someone who comes across, as "the way it is for me is the way it is for everyone." However, judicious and strategic use of self-disclosure builds trust. It conveys empathy by revealing that you have had (or have) your challenges too. Again, you are the ally, not the expert.

Any time you have an opportunity to make a difference
in this world and you don't, then you are
wasting your time on Earth.

—Roberto Clemente

My Own Story

Like many people I would experience muscle tension headaches from the tight muscles in my back. For many years my massage therapist, chiropractors and other had told me that strength training would help my occasional but persistent back problems immensely. However, I did not like strength training. I hated calisthenics. I was into aerobic conditioning and flexibility training through running, Yoga and Tai Chi. I was turned off by pumping iron.

I was well into my coaching career and a friend of mine and I were in the habit of meeting often at a local bagel shop. Before my eyes I watched him transform from a middle-aged guy with a pot belly into this amazingly strong, lean and vibrant man! I was intrigued to say the least. We had often talked about his career and family life challenges but his wellness lifestyle was an extremely positive factor that helped everything else in his life. He shared with me what he was doing to be suddenly so fit. He was following a well-structured diet and exercise program that was well researched and seemed to have a lot of validity to it. I was very curious.

I had coached many people who had engaged in one form or another of structured fitness/diet programs. Some programs were quite pre-packaged, others were self-administered following a book's instructions. I had never done any kind of program like that myself.

In my mid-fifties I embarked on unknown territory. With my friend's guidance, I began the same program. I bought the book and the accompanying materials. I began planning everything I ate and, most importantly, recorded everything that I actually did eat, six days a week. I began working out six days a week. My friend knew a lot about proper lifting technique and helped me to follow the program and include, for the first time, strength training into my exercise regiment. I stuck to it, and because of that, it worked!

Benefits for Me and For My Clients

The first one to benefit from the experience was me! I felt great! My energy level was much more constant throughout the day. I felt good about myself for losing ten pounds that all seemed to have been located around my waist, and certainly felt more attractive. I was clearly stronger and able to hike, paddle a canoe and lift portage loads easier. I also had to sheepishly admit that what the chiropractors and massage therapists had been telling me for years was true…strength training helped my back tremendously. I went through my first totally headache-free month in many years.

The others who benefited from my experience were my clients and students of wellness and wellness coaching. Before the new program I had been living a pretty good wellness lifestyle, exercising fairly regularly, but I had never engaged in any kind of a structured program.

Empathy for my clients who struggle with fitness programs and diets reached a new high. Suddenly I understood more from direct experience than I had been able to comprehend before. I knew that the experience of each of my clients was uniquely their own, but now I had more of a foothold in their world. It taught me many things about what that experience is like, and it taught me several principles that work to help someone lose weight and be fit.

Conscious Awareness Works

I realized that the awareness process of planning meals and then recording them was key. Unplanned meals for me had a tendency to be something quick and easy like white spaghetti pasta and bottled sauce, or a run to a restaurant. Planned meals were balanced, and more in line with things I really did like to eat. Recording them kept me honest, and kept the plan working.

Recording workouts in detail also helped me both stay regular and learn about this area of fitness that was new to me—strength training. I used solid principles from exercise physiology to guide my workouts and increased weights slowly, relying greatly on the principal of muscle development through adequate rest for the muscle groups affected.

Self-Perception

Probably the most powerful thing that the experience taught me came from the photographs. The program recommended that I take photographs of myself, just in a swimsuit, before the program, and afterwards. Mug shots of front, side and back views were brutally honest. I felt so bad about the digital pics that I took that I buried them somewhere in my computer where they would never show up accidentally on the screen.

When the ten weeks were up I took the second set of photos and examined them. I was disappointed in my results. Even though I had lost ten pounds, and more importantly, had lost almost ten per cent of my body fat, I still looked fat and out of shape. I was discouraged.

I looked for the before pictures and couldn't un-earth them from the depths of my hard drive. Having only the after pictures to look at, I focused in on the gut that was still there, the arms that had not transformed into guns, etc. Then, I finally found the before pictures and put them up side by side with the after pictures on my computer screen. My jaw dropped in astonishment. There was tremendous improvement evident.

Evident? It was obvious! I did look better. My back showed a lot of improvement, shifting from a weak looking structure holding up fairly broad shoulders, to a strong and healthy looking back. My gut was still there, but it had slimmed down! I realized how incredibly subjective the whole body image and self-perception experience is and how it can affect one's feelings. Of course I had worked over the years with many clients who struggled with these issues, but now I experienced first hand, what it was like. Looking in the mirror is ridiculous. We may as well look in a mirror at a carnival funhouse. Only when I had the objectivity of a camera lens did I see my improvement. No wonder my clients are so often discouraged, even when they do make progress!

Insuring Your Own Personal Wellness Foundation

Contrary to what one might imagine, not everyone who becomes a wellness coaching student is in stellar physical condition and optimal health. Not everyone in the wellness field runs marathons, meditates daily, eats a perfect diet, and climbs mountains on the weekends. We all tend, like our clients, to be incredibly—human! Our own wellness journeys teach us much that we can then apply to our coaching, but first of all they serve us ourselves.

Here are some quick guidelines for working on your own Personal Wellness Foundation.

1. Read and apply "The Ten Tenets of Wellness" to your own life. This sums up the basic principles for living your life well.

2. Work with a coach. This seems obvious, but it is important to not only buy into this concept and learn from it, but to benefit from it as well.

3. Value every aspect of your life: mind, body, spirit and environment. Many of us have learned to only value intellectual development. Embrace the aspect that you have been neglecting most.

4. Make sure your movement (exercise) includes all three areas: endurance, strength and flexibility. Do the things that challenge you, and that you tend to avoid.

5. Pay attention to current health research and decide what to apply from it to your own life. Constantly learn from trusted sources.

6. Increase connectedness in your life, in every way possible. Lubricate existing connections to friends, family and neighbors. If you are self-employed this is especially critical.

7. Make it about your personal growth! Get excited about continuing to grow as a person and much of the motivation to be well in every aspect of your life will follow.

8. Practice extreme self care. Enough with the taking care of everyone else to the exclusion of yourself! Others benefit the most from a healthy and happy you!

9. Write it down. Maintain a personal wellness journal, and use methods that allows you to keep track of your wellness efforts.

10. Move your body outdoors whenever possible. Make the natural world your ally.

11. Discover what centers you in your life and do more of it on a regular basis, be it reading, dancing, connecting with friends, gardening, hiking or other activity.

12. Remember you are not your work.

It is the call to service, giving our life over to something larger than ourselves, the call to become what we were meant to become – the call to achieve our vital design.

—Joe Jaworski
Synchronicity—The Inner Path of Leadership

Chapter 6

Creating the Alliance:
Let the Coaching Begin!

I have seen that in any great undertaking it is not enough
for a man to depend simply upon himself.

—**Lone Man** (Isna-la-wica)—Teton Sioux

Lone Man was a Teton Sioux who fought with Sitting Bull at the battle of Little Big Horn against Custer. His historical quote is ironic for a man of his name, yet it holds great wisdom. For a woman or man to simply depend upon themselves sounds ideal in many cultures. Self-sufficiency is a praiseworthy strength and I even include the concept in my "Ten Tenets of Wellness." Yet when we are faced with a truly great undertaking isn't it time for wisdom over strength alone? Today we would call it "working smarter, not harder."

Lone Man never considered taking on the Seventh Cavalry alone. When many of us attempt significant lifestyle change where we have failed before, it feels like the odds of success are about the same? It is a time for an ally, someone to help us move forward in a way we have not tried before.

Getting Clear On Coaching

One of the first tasks in wellness coaching is getting completely clear with your client about coaching and making sure it is a good fit for them. This might be done through an informal chat where you explain what coaching—and wellness coaching in particular—is and what it can do for a client. During this conversation you explore and really listen to the needs that your potential client has for services. Is coaching the right service for them at this time? If so, are you the right coach for them? If not you, then who might be? It's certainly about getting a good match formed where the client feels like they will be well served and progression towards their goals can be assured. A free mini-coaching session can be performed with the client at this time to give them a taste of what coaching is and contrast it with other helping experiences they have had.

If the client has come to see you in another capacity that you perform (wellness educator, nurse, fitness trainer, etc.), then introducing wellness coaching as another service that you can offer to help the client also requires clarity. Seek a mutual agreement that derives from the client understanding of what coaching is, how it works, and what it can do for them. Distinguish between the services that are part of your other role and the services of your coaching role. This is especially important when your non-coaching role is treatment or consultation oriented. When wellness professionals become more coach-like, they no longer just enroll, inform and educate their clients, they take the journey with them, by their sides. They accompany the client as their professional ally.

When you step into the role of coach and co-create an alliance to work together, the client needs to be aware of, and in agreement with, their own role as coachee. Especially in the area of wellness coaching you may find your clients, who are looking for ways to improve their lifestyle, still want you to take primary responsibility for this task. They may still be operating on the prescribe and treat mindset that they are used to, and that you have worked hard to shift out of.

Who's Responsible for What?

One of the absolute best questions to pose to a coaching client is "Who's responsible for what?" This is a great question for the client who is working through a conflict in the workplace, and an excellent question for all sorts of partners (business, marital, etc.) to be clear on. It is also a key question for wellness coaching.

One of the benefits of the coach approach that wellness professionals get really excited about is that it shifts responsibility for their own health and wellbeing back onto the client. Wellness professionals suddenly feel free of the burden of having to come up with all the answers for their client. By requiring their client to make their own effort coaches are not shirking their work and the client will benefit more from that approach. They've even learned how to deal with the clients who cry "Just tell me what to do!" by honoring their frustration, patiently explaining the benefits of an approach where the client finds their own answers and elaborating on how the coach can, and will, be of support.

Gaining buy-in from your client around the concept of self-responsibility for their own health may not be an overnight accomplishment. It is not about who's to blame for the state of one's health, but it is about the client's acceptance of responsibility for shifting their present lifestyle in such a way as to improve their health and reduce their risks. When clients give up the stance of the victim and embrace their own power to improve their lives, real progress begins.

You can pave the way towards such full acceptance of responsibility by working out with the client, in very concrete terms, who's responsible for what in the coaching alliance. Most coaches use agreement forms that spell out the details of the coaching arrangements. Appointment times, cancellation policies, fees and other details, are all spelled out in writing. As we'll see in later chapters, the coach also works with the client and their challenges and goals around the concept of accountability in a system of very clear agreements. (See the appendix)

We make all sorts of assumptions because we don't have the courage to ask questions.

—**Don Miguel Ruiz,** *The Four Agreements*

Agreements vs. Expectations

To be more coach-like when working with clients, be aware of which agreements have been made (and which have not), and be very aware of what expectations are being operated upon.

- Expectations are much like assumptions. We expect (assume) that Larry will know the right thing to do. We expect (assume) that Mary knows how she is supposed to follow up after our meeting.

- Expectations are much like wishing and hoping. We hope that Larry does his job the way we instructed him.

- Unmet expectations are very disappointing. The more we expect, the more we may be disappointed.

- Unmet expectations are very hard to confront. Failure to communicate the expectation properly will most likely result in someone being blamed instead of real responsibility being taken.

- Agreements clarify the question of "Who's responsible for what?"

- Agreements need to be fashioned continually even when it seems laborious to do so. Writing them down may help.

- Agreements work best when they are "true agreements," that is, the agreement is reached mutually.

- Broken agreements are easy to confront. "I thought we had an agreement that you would do_____ by_____."

- Clearly-stated agreements that seem impossible to meet can be re-negotiated with more ease than expectations or ambiguous agreements.

Expect nothing. Be prepared for anything.

—Samurai saying

"Expect nothing. Be prepared for anything." This does not mean expect nothing to happen. It means do not have any expectations. It means to expect only what is agreed upon to happen. Approach each person and each situation without assumptions or expectations. Make clear agreements.

Coaching pioneer Thomas Leonard was fond of saying: "Give up all hope . . . but have faith." Wishing and hoping don't get the job done. Faith in yourself and others (who have earned your trust) and, perhaps in, shall we say, "something greater" does work!

Permission

The coach is aware of what a coaching relationship needs to look like. The client may not be as familiar with it. To proceed and attain agreements as a coach you need to operate using the process of permission over and over again. Whitworth, et.al., *Co-Active Coaching* (2011), call permission the heart of the intake session. They see all actions being filtered through this process, which continually honors the client. Doing so helps the client realize that they are the ones in charge and that you are working for them. Clients learn their role is not that of student or unquestioning patient, but rather as decision maker, the captain of their soul and master of their fate.

Coaching language is permeated with permission. Continually ask your client "May I ask about . . . ?" "Can we explore this further?" "Would you like to look deeper into this area, or not?" "May I make a suggestion?" "Would you like to hear about some resources I know of in this area?" Permission continually honors the client and their own ability to help themselves. It also really helps you to stay within the mindset of ally, not expert.

The Foundation Session: Two Time-Tracks for Wellness Coaching

Much of the literature on coaching and psychotherapy is written based on the private practice or clinic model of lengthy appointments. The "fifty minute hour" of counseling and therapy is quite standard. In coaching most scenarios describe a one or two hour foundation session, followed by either half-hour appointments (most commonly on a weekly or four-a-month basis), or even hour-long appointments.

Wellness coaches who either have their own business, or are working with organizations as an out-sourced wellness coach may work on the same time model. There are some situations where an on-staff wellness coach may have this much time available to work with clients, but not often. Frequently either the wellness professional doing wellness coaching as part of what they do or the wellness coach in a corporate or healthcare setting has a very brief amount of time with their client. Fifteen to twenty minutes may be the maximum contact time they get with a client at any one time. To honor the reality of these two different time situations, I will present two different approaches to working with wellness coaching clients. There is much overlap in the models because the basic concepts used in both are the same. Time availability and how to focus the coaching quickly are the main differences.

Sample Agreement

Client name: _____

Address: _____

Phone #: _____

Email: _____

Initial Term _____ Months   From _____ through _____

This fee is _____ per month and my method of payment will be _____

Session day: _____ Session time: _____ Session length: _____ Sessions per month: _____

Referred by: _____

Other: _____

Protocol:
1. Client calls the coach at the scheduled time.
2. Client pays the coaching fees in advanced.
3. Client pays for long-distance charges, if any.

1. As a client, I understand that I am fully responsible for my well-being during my coaching call, including my choices and decisions. I am aware that I can choose to discontinue coaching at any time. I recognize that coaching is not psychotherapy or any form of medical treatment, and that professional referrals will be given if needed.
2. I understand that "life coaching" or "wellness coaching" is a relationship I have with my coach that is designed to facilitate the creation/development of personal, professional, and/or business goals and to develop and carry out a strategy/plan for achieving those goals.
3. I understand that life/wellness coaching is a comprehensive process that may involve all areas of my life, including work, finances, health, relationships, educations and recreation. I acknowledge that deciding how to handle these issues and implement my choices is exclusively my responsibility.
4. I understand that life/wellness coaching does not treat mental disorders as described by the American Psychiatric Association. I understand that life/wellness coaching is not a substitute for counseling, psychotherapy, psychoanalysis, mental health care or substance abuse treatment, and I will not use it in place of any form of therapy.
5. I promise that if I am currently in therapy or otherwise under the care of a mental health professional, that I have consulted with this person regarding the advisability of working with a life/wellness coach and that this person is aware my decision to proceed with the life coaching relationship.
6. I understand that information will be held as confidential unless I state otherwise, in writing, except as required by law.
7. I understand that certain topics may be anonymously shared with other wellness coaching professionals for training or consultation purposes.
8. I understand that wellness coaching is not to be used in lieu of professional advice. I will seek professional guidance for legal, medical, financial, business, spiritual, or other matters. I understand that all decisions in these areas are exclusively mine, and I acknowledge that my decisions and my actions regarding them are my responsibility.

I have read and agreed to the above.

_____   _____
            Client Signature   Date

Reproducible Worksheet Masters are available for purchase on CD ROM from Whole Person Associates, 101 W. 2nd St., Suite 203, Duluth, MN 55802, 800-247-6789, www.wholeperson.com.

FIGURE 6.1

Sample Client Policies and Procedures

Welcome to coaching as my client. I look forward to working with you. There are a few guidelines that I expect clients to maintain in order for the relationship to work. If you have any question, please call me.

Fee: Clients pay me on time unless prior arrangements have been made. Payment maybe made by check or credit card.

Procedure: My clients call on time. Come to the call with updates, progress, and current challenges. Let me know what you want to work on , and be ready to be coached. Make copies of the enclosed/attached client prep form and email a completed form to before each call. The agenda is client generated and coach-supported.

Calls/ Sessions: Our agreement includes a set amount of calls. If you or I are on vacation, we will spend more time before you/I leave and after you/I return.

Changes: My clients give me 24 hours notice if they have to cancel or reschedule a call. If you have an emergency, we will work around it. Otherwise a missed call is not made up.

Extra Time: You may call me between our scheduled sessions if you need "spot coaching", have a problem, or can't wait to share a success with me. (You can also email or text me) I enjoy delivering this extra level of service. I do not bill for additional time of this type, but ask that you keep the calls short. when you leave a message let me know if you would like a call back or if you are just sharing.

Problems: I want you to be satisfied with our relationship. If I ever say or do something that upsets you or doesn't feel right, please bring it to my attention. As your coach, I am 100% committed to you being powerful, successful and to you having the life you want.

A Must: It is necessary for the client to be active participant in the coaching for it to be successful. You have hired a coach to help you do things differently. If you choose to not use the coaching and keep doing what you have always done, you will get the same results you have always received.

Reproducible Worksheet Masters are available for purchase on CD ROM from Whole Person Associates, 101 W. 2nd St., Suite 203, Duluth, MN 55802, 800-247-6789, www.wholeperson.com.

FIGURE 6.2

Track One—The Conventional Time Coaching Model

Once you have established clear agreements about your coaching it's time to launch the coaching process through your Foundation Session. Intake sounds too clinical for the first coaching meeting. In this session you are building the alliance together by laying the foundation of your professional relationship together. Some coaches call this the exploration or discovery session.

The Foundation Session Is About:

- Exploration
- Listening deeply to the client's story and honoring it through acknowledgement.
- Grounding the coach in the world of the client.
- Building trust.

- Determining what works best for coaching this particular client.

- Getting clear on what the client is asking for in the coaching relationship.

- Evaluating the client's readiness for change on key areas they want to work on.

- Co-creating an initial wellness plan based on areas of focus and readiness. Sometimes this comes later, after more adequate exploration.

- Getting the client started with initial action-steps for which they are prepared.

The ideal format is for the coach to have the client complete a welcome packet (see appendix) and perhaps a wellness assessment tool (online or paper) before the foundation session takes place. The coach and client then schedule either two contiguous hours for the foundation session, or two one-hour appointments within the first one or two weeks to go over the information you have gathered and do the foundational work.

The foundation session should have a comfortable flow to it where the coach and client are meeting each other as equals and getting acquainted. Differing in intent from a casual or even business-like connection, the wellness coaching relationship is started with the conscious intention that it be an alliance designed to help the client improve their lifestyle.

Foundation Session Road Map

Within the flow of interaction the coach follows a road map that makes sure important processes are completed. While you might create your own content to such a map, certain areas need to be considered. These would include:

- *Connect with your client.* Relate with genuineness, honesty and sincerity.

- *Get on the same page.* Inquire about the best way to coach this person. Offer them choices and options. Help them see what coaching entails and what might work best with them.

- *Begin your exploration together.* Ask directly what they would like to focus on in coaching.

- *Get a horizon-to-horizon view.* Use a simple tool like The Wheel of Life to help the client get a complete view of balance and fulfillment in their entire life.

- *Clarify values.* Through questions, conversation, and possibly exercises, help the client to clarify what is important to them, what gives them meaning and purpose in life.

- *Take stock.* Help the client to recognize and acknowledge strengths they possess and where they receive support for a healthier way of living. What are they aware of (both within themselves, and in their environment) that is working for them and against themselves? How ready are they for change?

- *Co-create an initial wellness plan.* While we will work more completely on an Integrated Wellness Plan in later sessions, the client needs a place to start, an initial direction to take. Doing so capitalizes on their motivation to begin their journey of change.

  Based upon your exploration so far, help your client to select Areas of Focus that they are ready to work on. Within each Area of Focus help them determine at least one initial goal they want to reach. Then to begin their work on that goal help them determine an action step, or steps that they are "ready, willing and able" to make a commitment to work on.

INITIAL WELLNESS PLAN ⇨ AREA(S) OF FOCUS
⇨ GOAL(S) ⇨ ACTION STEP(S)

FIGURE 6.3

  Agree upon "indicators of success," that is criteria that will allow your client to have a measure of success that they can work towards accomplishing.

- *Secure an agreement* of accountability.

- *Leave the client knowing* exactly what to do next, and exactly how to prepare for the next session.

- *Leave them with an inquiry*—something to ponder about themselves and their way of living.

Track Two—The Limited Time Coaching Model

In the situation where a wellness professional is individualizing the wellness services that they provide through using wellness coaching and/or wellness coaching skills, time is often limited. Some common scenarios may look like this:

- An employee is given a wellness/health assessment (usually an HRA—health risk assessment), and a follow-up session is provided. The wellness professional usually has somewhere between 15 and 55 minutes with this person, with 20-30 minutes being most common.

- An employee is attracted to wellness coaching services that are offered as an aspect of a larger wellness program offered by their employer. These are usually time limited and often focused on specific challenges.

- An employee may be referred for wellness coaching by the medical/health program of the organization, but the system only allows for very brief sessions.

In the role of the wellness professional you are faced with many of the same tasks outlined above, connecting with the client, building trust, etc. Your real challenge is that you need to do this in much less time, and yet still be effective.

A Key Skill From Coaching For Time Limited Wellness Coaching: Laser Coaching

The profession of coaching has developed some skills that are more central to personal coaching and serve this time-limited situation well. Thomas Leonard, a founder of the coaching movement, liked to urge coaches to use laser coaching. The key here is for you to maintain empathy and compassion, and yet cut through the client's story and maintain laser-like focus without any distracting tangents being allowed. The more masterful coach can acknowledge the client's experience and help them feel heard, yet will continually guide the client to stay on the subject at hand, get to the point (which can be fact or feeling), and help the client assess what action they are ready to take (or not).

Often the content of the client's story is not as important as how they felt about it, or what they have concluded about it in their lives. There may be a very long and drawn out story about how someone became overweight that a client feels compelled to share. Your client may actually not feel so much of a need to share it anymore (having done so with many others before you), but may assume that you want to hear the entire tale. You may have to interrupt this process and, after acknowledging their experience and its importance to them, urge them to move ahead in the story to the most recent chapters. Let them know that you really care about how their experience is affecting them now. Ask powerful questions that help them focus on what is important in the present.

In the field of Gestalt therapy the emphasis is not on the past, but on the here and now. Borrowing from this way of working with people, we help our clients to "presentify" their experience. We acknowledge that we cannot do a thing about the past, what happened was real, and the key is how the person feels about it, how it affects them, and what they are aware of about it in the present.

> Client: "My Mother was so critical! Every time I would try something new she always pointed out how I did it wrong."

> Coach: "That must have been terribly difficult to grow up with such constant criticism."

> Client: "Yeah, she used to do it about everything! The clothes I wore, my performance in high school band, my friends, and of course my weight!"

> Coach: "So how does your experience of your Mother's criticism back then affect your efforts at weight loss today? How does it get in the way now?"

> Client: "You know, it really does. When I begin a new weight loss program I have this nagging feeling that I'm going to fail...right from the start! It's like I can hear her telling me it won't work."

Forgiveness is giving up all hope for a better past.

—Jack Kornfield

The Foundation Session (Time-Limited Model) Is About:

- Showing evidence that you are listening to the client's story and honoring it through acknowledgement.

- Grounding (the coach) in the world of the client.

- Building trust quickly and genuinely.

- Determining what works best for coaching this particular client.

- Clearly establishing what the client is asking for in the coaching relationship.

- Conveying to the client what the coaching relationship can look like, given the time- limited nature of this specific coaching situation.

- Evaluating the client's readiness for change on the key areas they want to work on.

- Co-creating an initial wellness plan based on areas of focus and readiness for change.

- Getting the client started with initial action-steps for which they are prepared.

As you can see, much of the same work needs to be done, but in a much shorter time frame. The reality is that the same degree of depth and even accuracy about what really needs to be worked on will be less likely to be accomplished. This is one of the trade-offs that comes with the time-limited territory. It is not a true substitute for the broader and deeper work that the conventional coaching model will bring.

Foundation Session Road Map—Time Limited Model

- *Connect with your client.* Relate with genuineness, honesty and sincerity.

- *Give the client a quick introduction* to the structure of your time together and how it can/will be used. Share the responsibility for keeping track of the time during the session.

- *Begin your exploration together.* Ask directly what they would like to focus on in the session.

- *Bring the session into focus.* If they have completed a tool like an HRA, begin to review it. Start by asking what the experience of taking it was like. * *Get welcome packet and basic assessment information online or by fax prior to the foundational session to save time and allow you time to review before the session.*

- *Take stock.* Help the client to recognize and acknowledge strengths they possess and where they receive support for a healthier way of living. What are they aware of (both within themselves, and in their environment) that is working for them and against themselves? How ready are they for change?

- *Make it more coach-like.* Explain to the client how you can be more of a coach with them, instead of only providing treatment or education, and what that can look like.

- *Co-create an initial wellness plan.* In a time-limited Foundation Session, the client still needs to leave feeling like they have a basic plan. A more complete wellness plan will be developed later, but for now help them to establish at least one or two Areas of Focus, a Goal within each and one Action Step that they are ready to commit to working on between now and the time of the next appointment. Even if it is very simple, help your client feel like they are engaged in this coaching process, that their journey has begun.

- *Secure an agreement* of accountability.

- *Leave the client knowing* exactly what to do next, and exactly how to prepare for the next session and securing a time for that to happen.

- *Leave them with an inquiry*—something to ponder about themselves and their way of living.

Trust

What allows a client to walk into a room, or pick up a phone, and start trusting someone? Establishing trust is central to the coaching relationship. As a wellness coach, what do you have going for you,to help establish trust from the beginning? What do you have to do to earn and grow that trust?

Trust men and they will be true to you; treat them greatly,
and they will show themselves great.

—Ralph Waldo Emerson

Trust is often difficult to wrap one's arms around. What is it really? How can we define it? Merriam-Webster's Dictionary defines it as "assured reliance on the character, strength, or truth of someone or something." The question now becomes what is present in the character of someone that allows us to assign that assured reliance? One way of breaking it down is to look for the consistent presence of integrity, competence and compassion.

As a wellness coach you first convey integrity by simply being who you are. Don Miguel Ruiz (*The Four Agreements*) calls it "being impeccable with your word." You speak the truth, you say what you mean, and mean what you say. You are reliable and predictable. You can be counted on. You are the ally you purport to be.

You also convey integrity by your level of professionalism. Your clients will be more likely to trust a healthcare professional (the good side of the "white coat effect"), and a truly professional coach who comes across as well trained and preferably is certified in that training. Integrity is also implied by the coach handling their business in a professional business-like way with a business-like (yet caring) appearance.

Competence will also show through in the actions of the well-trained and professional coach. When coaches demonstrate the competencies listed by the ICF as central to the profession of coaching (see appendix), clients know they are in good hands and trust increases as the relationship goes on.

Compassion is the heart and soul of coaching. It is a human being-to-human being experience of acceptance, caring and understanding. Even if we do not agree with the other person's actions, we accept them and reach within ourselves to attempt to understand the other person's experience. Compassion is complete when we find a way to convey it to the other person.

For someone who must struggle to share compassion with others, choosing coaching profession is about the most incongruent career fit there is. If we are not being compassionate, are we being judgmental?

It is hard to tread some kind of neutral space between the two. Empathy and compassion is how we move out of judgment. They are how we train our psyche to avoid being judgmental.

When we come into contact with the other person,
our thoughts and actions should express our mind of
compassion, even if that person says and does things that
are not easy to accept. We practice in this way until we see
clearly that our love is not contingent upon the other person
being lovable.

—Thich Nhat Hanh

Everyone has trust issues. We cannot control, and are not responsible for the trust issues of others that make forming an alliance more challenging. All we can do is live our lives as the kind of person others can put their trust in. Trust is partly about doing (our consistent and reliable actions), but largely about being. The more we coach from the centered place of who we truly are, the more trustworthy we appear.

Foundational Coaching Skills

You have a client who is seeking ways to improve their life and their lifestyle. You've connected and co-created a coaching alliance that has you both excited about change. Now what do you do?

You are making good use of your basic coaching skills and you have taken it one step further into the realm of wellness coaching. Our purpose here is not to duplicate the already great training that is out there on basic coaching skills. Understanding and developing competency in the ICF Coaching Core Competencies (see appendix) are critical to the development of a professional coach. On the foundational level though, because of its importance, I would like to share more on the importance of listening and using more powerful questions.

Giving Evidence Of Listening

Seek first to understand, then to be understood.

—Stephen Covey

A central part of the training that anyone in any kind of human service receives is about the importance of listening. In the conflict training that I developed twenty years ago, I saw how vital it is that people in conflict feel they are truly being heard. A perception that they are being dismissed or not really being listened to, escalates the conflict. People speak louder (as though you truly are not hearing the sounds they are making), get angrier, and move closer to violence. When people feel they are being heard, they calm down, speak softer and are more reasonable. The conflict usually de-escalates. When people talk about their health and wellbeing, really personal and vital topics for them, you need to listen with professional skill.

When we need to tell our story, we want to be heard and we want to know that we are being heard. When my dog, or a deer I see in the woods listens to sounds I am making I can tell because their ears move. Since it would be possible for me to sit in front of you motionless and speechless, and yet have my ears work perfectly, taking in every sound you make, how do you know that I am really listening? We have all experienced conversations where our "listener" was making good eye contact while their thoughts were miles away.

There is much more to listening than having my ear drums vibrate with your sound waves. Am I getting it? Am I understanding and comprehending what you are saying? How do you know that you are, in fact, making a connection? Well, I have to give you evidence that I really am listening.

Giving evidence is about observable behavior. Your client needs to be able to see and hear evidence that you are not only absorbing sounds, you are really hearing them. We do this in two primary ways, non-verbal and verbal behavior.

Evidence of effective listening non-verbal behaviors include good eye contact, appropriate and naturally changing facial expression, open posture and natural, relaxed movement. During a face-to-face, rather than teleconference coaching session, you have the opportunity to build trust and faith with your client by evidencing good non-verbal coaching listening behavior. It's your chance to show them that you are really with them.

The words you say that can be transcribed on paper are your vocal behavior. The rest is non-verbal. Make good use of your voice to engender trust, sincerity, self-disclosure, and commitment. If you tend to have a soft voice, this is a time to pump up the volume. If you tend to be loud, use your voice volume very, very consciously. Tone, inflection, accentuation, and that elusive conveyance of sincerity, are all key to demonstrating that you are really with your client every step of the way.

Verbal Evidence of Listening

When I reiterate to you the essence of what you just said, then you know that I am listening to you well. The good ol' basic coaching skills of paraphrasing, reflection of feeling, and summarization really shine here. Using them shows your client that you are tracking well with them. You give evidence that you not only are hearing the words correctly, but that you get the meaning, the feeling, of what your client is saying. As simple as this sounds, it is of paramount importance. Listening on many levels and doing it well, then giving evidence to your client that this is what you are doing, builds the coaching alliance perhaps better than anything else. Continuing to give this evidence continues and deepens the relationship and the effectiveness of the coaching.

The Great Good Spirit gave us two ears and one mouth so
we would listen twice as much as we speak.

—**Shawnee** (Native American) saying

Active Listening Skills Used in Coaching

Skillful listeners help people feel "heard"! The client who has a great listener for a coach not only feels understood, they have their feelings and thoughts validated. They feel like someone understands their struggles and challenges, their hopes and regrets. They have someone who celebrates and acknowledges every bit of progress they make. They also have someone who catches things that they miss. They have someone who acts like a special mirror that helps reduce their own blind-spots.

There are specific skills that great coaches use to deliver profound listening: Paraphrase & Restatement; Reflection of Feeling; Use of Silence; Relying on Intuition; Request for Clarification; Acknowledgement; Summarization.

Active Listening Skills used in Coaching

Paraphrasing / Restatement — stating back to the person the essence of what they have just said; reassures the person that they are being heard and understood; allows them to realize what they said; gives them the opportunity to clarify their true meaning. Clients are often surprised to realize what they just said. It also provides continual "evidence of listening." Example of paraphrasing:

> *Client: "The workload is getting crazy at my job. They've cut back on personnel and we all have to cover the gap."*
>
> *Coach: "So, with all the cutbacks, work has gotten unmanageable."*

- Restatement is when we simply repeat the person's words verbatim in a tone of "checking it out" with them.

Reflection of Feeling — getting at the meaning behind the words and feeding it back to the person; mirroring back to the person more of the feeling that is present and being experienced rather than content. This helps the client get across what they are often really trying to communicate with all of their words. They are essentially saying "I feel this way, please understand!" It also helps clients get in touch with what they actually are feeling at a deeper level. It takes the coaching to a deeper and often more effective level. This is not the same as interpretation. You are offering to the client your estimation of what feeling you are observing and reflecting back to the client what you are seeing. Examples: *"It sounds like this must be really difficult for you." "You seem really excited..." "What I hear is perhaps you are worried about this."*

Use of Silence — wait about a moment or two before responding; an extended silence will prompt the client to think more about the issue and add detail; it lets the story unfold; it puts the responsibility back on the person for them to develop the dialogue. Using a balance of active engagement and silence allows the coach to let the coaching be more client-directed, and often allows for deepening. This is particularly effective right after the client makes a very powerful statement. It allows them to go where they need to go, rather than where a question of yours might have taken them.

Relying On Your Intuition or your gut feeling and share it; another form of reflection; always offer this tentatively allowing the person to correct you if you're off target. Use this skill sparingly but learn to trust it more and more. Example: *"Joe, tell me if I'm off base here, but I'm getting the feeling that..."*

Requesting Clarification — asking for elaboration on anything you're unsure about or anything that leaves room for error; allows the client to continue and deepen their exploration; reassures the person that you want to understand them completely; avoids assumptions. Examples: *"Tell me more..." "What about this..." "Can you tell me what you mean by..."* Much more neutral than a question.

Acknowledging — Share with the individual the value of who they are and the validity of their experience, as well as what they did. Examples: *"I want to acknowledge the sensitivity you showed when you spoke with your spouse about the conflict over what foods to prepare that you two were having."* Clients often don't "give themselves credit" for what they have accomplished. The sharp coach notices and acknowledges every bit of success.

Summarization – Review in a concise way what has been expressed and experienced in the coaching so far. Do this at the end of every coaching session, but also periodically throughout the session itself. It is kind of like an author of a long novel refreshing the reader's understanding of the plot. This also helps the client stay very focused and on task. It helps at the end of a session to clarify what was covered, and what has been agreed to for next steps.

Using Powerful Questions In Coaching

The Elements of Powerful Questions
In order for a question to be powerful, it should:

- Open the individual up to possibilities

- Not presume an answer

- Promote deep thinking

- Be in positive terms

- Be delivered in an appropriate tone of voice

It is important that questions are not leading. The coach needs to be in a centered place in order for this to happen. Stay in the present – don't anticipate what to say next or attempt to hand out a solution of yours.

Don't be attached to the outcome. We love to say that the coach is "In The Inquiry" instead of "In The Question." By this we mean that the coach doesn't care if the client actually answers "their" question, instead they are excited about how questions help catalyze the whole process of exploration for the client. Be more concerned about the person's experience than the details and the drama of the situation at hand. Work from the assumption that our natural state is curious. Support your client to see their own answer instead of giving them your answer

Use questions sparingly. Use your other coaching communications more of the time. (paraphrasing, reflective listening, etc.) Change questions into requests like *"Tell me more about..."*

Many new coaches believe that they have to continuously ask their clients questions and they often forget to use the other Active Listening Skills (paraphrase, request for clarification, etc.). Coaching is a very client- centered process and we want our clients to have enough freedom to talk about what is most important to them. We want our questions to aid in that process and not be so directive that our clients have to go where we want them to go in order to answer our questions. Mix it up! Pepper the coaching conversation with powerful questions, but use the Active Listening Skills at least 50% of the time, if not more.

In wellness coaching I have seen coaches who are enthusiastic about particular approaches to wellness (following certain diets, particular exercise routines, or meditation practices) try to "guide" their clients to conclusions that they (the coach) want them to reach. The coach's questions lead, and frankly manipulate, the client to conclude that the coach's favorite wellness regiment is golden answer they have been searching for. This is not coaching! It is, as we stated, manipulation.

Using Open-Ended Questions

Closed Questions require limited short answers from the client.
- *Did you run today?* Yes!
- Do you like to exercise? No!

Open-ended Questions require the client to look inside and reference their thoughts, feelings and experiences to give an answer.
- What activities do you like to do?
- How do you feel when you walk on a regular basis?

Forget "Why?" Questions!

Your clients have probably been asking themselves "Why?" for a very long time and are still perplexed. They don't need their coach to ask them *"Why?"* again. 80-90% of the time the answer will be *"I don't know."* Believe your client! They don't know. Why questions also can feel like accusations. *Why don't you exercise more? Why do you continue to eat deep-fried food when you're trying to lose weight?* Clients become defensive and coaching can grind to a halt.

Instead of *"Why?"* questions, change them to *"How?"*, *"What?"*, *"When?"*, *"Where?"* questions.

How often do you go out walking?

When do you have the opportunity to exercise?

How do you feel when you eat a lighter dinner?

What would be an area you want to focus on right now?

The Key To Exploration With Questions

Once you've gotten beyond getting acquainted and have built the coaching alliance by becoming familiar with your client's life (asking them questions about their living situation, work, health, etc.) the questions cease to be "for you"...they are "for" your client! Your job as a coach is to facilitate your client's own exploration of themselves and their life. **Pose questions for your clients to ask themselves.** Create powerful questions for the client to consider and reflect upon. Let go of playing detective and be a real facilitator of change and growth.

Chapter 7

Charting the Course of Change: Wellness Mapping 360°™ Part I

The most fundamental aggression to ourselves, the most
fundamental harm we can do to ourselves, is to remain
ignorant by not having the courage and the respect to look at
ourselves honestly and gently.

—Pema Chodrin
When Things Fall Apart

Wellness coaches help their clients to see their health and wellbeing as part of an infinite and incredibly interconnected web. Our wellness is determined not just by ideas we have, or information we are aware of, but by every aspect of that web. When we tug on one strand, the vibration is felt in the entire web.

I often explain to my new clients that during the course of our coaching we will at times roll up our sleeves and put our elbows on the table and really focus on one particular thing. At other times, we will shove ourselves away from the table and go out and get into a hot-air balloon, where we will rise up into the sky and look at their life from horizon to horizon, three hundred and sixty degrees.

In the medical model it is easy to slip into an analytic, atomistic, sequential process that narrows down a wealth of information into a diagnosis. Conventional medicine today is starting to realize that mere symptom reduction diagnosis and treatment are inadequate. The tremendous surge in the use of integrative medicine approaches in Europe, North America and elsewhere, is evidence that the public sees increasing value in methods that work with the whole person. Since wellness is a holistic concept, wellness coaching, by its very definition is holistic.

In the next chapters we will look at ways to help our clients improve their lifestyle behavior by fashioning a path through the huge landscape of wellness and health. To guide them and you on that journey we have developed a process or a model of wellness coaching we call Wellness Mapping 360°™.

Wellness Mapping 360°™

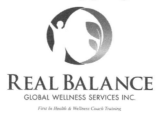

REAL BALANCE
GLOBAL WELLNESS SERVICES INC.
First In Health & Wellness Coach Training

Assessment & Exploration

Never assume the obvious is true.

—William Safire

Sometimes our clients know exactly what they want to work on, and sometimes getting clear about it is your starting point. Remember the "You Are Here" marks on maps in downtown areas or shopping malls? Every journey has to start from somewhere, but some of our clients come to us precisely because they know a journey is needed, but they really aren't sure what port they are setting sail from. To begin our voyage of discovery and exploration of wellness, we have to be very clear about where we are from the start.

Groundedness

In many spiritual traditions the purpose of ceremony is to ground you and orient you so that you have a solid sense of where you are to begin your journey to higher places. The coaching relationship itself helps to do this. As your client tells you their story, answers your powerful questions, and completes your assessment instruments, they do so only partly to provide you with information. They do so to hear themselves, and sometimes they are surprised at what they discover themselves saying. The foundation session(s) helps them organize their thinking and helps them review and take stock of their lives. This grounds them in the present moment, taking the focus off the desired outcome that perhaps brought them through the coaching door and brings them to the here and now

Coaches believe their clients. When your client speaks you are there to listen and work with them, not to judge them. Since you are not in a treatment situation, you are not there to "figure out what is really going on." Your job is not to dig for the truth. It is to create the container in which the client feels safe enough to reveal the truth, to you, and to themselves.

In therapy I would often find clients would come in with what I called an "admission ticket." Their "ticket" was some sort of issue that was less fearful to discuss. As trust was developed they often felt safe enough to talk about the more serious, underlying issue. In coaching I don't sit in suspicion. I do, however, never make an assumption that what I've heard is the entire story. Likewise, I never assume that every molehill is yearning to become a mountain.

The Value of Self-Exploration

Requests from clients need to be taken at face value. If your client says they are here to lose weight, here's the diet, here's the exercise program, let's go, what are you to do? They just might be so ready to change that all they need is some of the support and accountability aspects of coaching. They may also be doing what they think they should do, or what they have always done before (and usually failed at). You don't want to throw cold water on their enthusiasm, but you might also invite them to take a good look at where they are right now before they launch into their program.

The wellness journey, or quest, begins like any other classic quest, with self-knowledge. The coaching process can be the rare oasis where the client has complete permission to take a deeper look at their self. The style of wellness coaching that I teach emphasizes motivation, not information. Many of your clients will have a fair to excellent understanding about what they need to do to be well. Helping them understand their own motivation, and the lack thereof, is a true value the coach can offer.

It may be very tempting to stay in the diagnose and treat mindset and quickly set up a behavioral coach-knows-best program. When we remind ourselves to stay in the coaching mindset of the wellness ally, we shift into a mode of facilitation and allowing, of assisting our client on their journey.

Allow your client adequate time, to the degree you can, to tell their story. You are not there to be therapist-like or priest-like, but instead to be a witness. Your professional level of listening, your very genuine and human compassion, your challenging coach nature, will help them feel acknowledged, validated and whole. The bonus for your client is that this very basic human process helps them fight their own inner critic, their own demons, that have been sabotaging their previous attempts at lifestyle change. This strengthening process is like getting in shape physically before you head off to climb the 14,000 foot peak.

We shall not cease from exploration and the end of all our exploring will be to arrive where we started . . . and know the place for the first time.

—T.S. Eliot

Tools for Exploration

Part of the power of coaching is that it does not just take place for one fifty-minute hour a week. It is an ongoing process for the client beyond the time in person or on the phone with the coach. Encourage your client to explore themselves in greater breadth and depth by using a number of other tools.

1. Journaling. When you sit around and think you engage in one type of cognitive process. When you speak with me you engage in yet another cognitive process. When you sit down and write, you engage in still another cognitive process. Why not use all three?

Encourage your client to journal in a way that fits for them. Secure a commitment from them (if they are up for it) as to how many times a week they will journal. Usually a commitment to write every single day is a set-up for self-failure. Committing to only once or twice a week probably deserves a challenge from the coach to examine what they truly would benefit most from.

2. Solo Time. If your client seems to have little time to reflect, perhaps they need to literally get away from it all. There is a rich tradition through history and all around the world that encourages the seeking soul to spend some time alone and away from business-as-usual. Christ's forty days in the wilderness, the Australian Bushman's walk about, the Native American vision quest, are all examples of processes that call upon solo time for insight, and often, breakthroughs.

There are profound guided experiences that your client might want to sign on for (see resources section). There are also ways in which a client may want to engineer some time away from work/home that are safe, and practical for them. Coach them through the process of planning and carrying out such a personal self-exploration process. (See "Living the Ten Tenets of Wellness" in Chapter Two.)

3. Bibliocoaching. What we used to call bibliotherapy now serves us in the personal growth arena as well. Coach your client through the process of selecting and following through on reading (yes, there's the value of a coach!), several titles that match their interest and the questions they hold for themselves. Sometimes good books on the very process of change, such as *Taming Your Gremlin* and *The Way We're Working Isn't Working*, can contain great insights. I find myself making extraordinary use of the Don Miguel Ruiz book *The Four Agreements*.

Some books may be more for wellness information, but in this exploration phase, books that point the way into self-exploration/self-discovery are very valuable. Ask permission to make suggestions if your client has no idea of where to start, or sit down and do some exploration online with them.

4. Life Review. Another tool to offer is the life review process. You might start with a time-line of the client's life that indicates from the date of birth onward, the significant events in the client's life. Make a yearly indicator across the timeline to the present, leaving the end open for the future. Then have your client enter on the timeline the events that occurred in their life at the time they happened. Ask them to write down what they learned from going through the experiences.

- How did you grow from it?

- What ways of living and coping did you adopt from it?

- Was your adopted behavior something that worked then, but doesn't serve you now?

Don't get into the paralysis of analysis. Support them in avoiding self-criticism and regret. Focus on how the person became who they are and how it affects them in the present moment.

Richard Bach in his little classic *Illusions* likes to say that everything we experience in life is either something we are learning from, or something we are just enjoying! Help your client in their exploration process realize what they are continuing to learn.

5. Quieting Practice. The process of change and self-exploration, insight and understanding requires patience. Sometimes it is like the old Japanese rice farmer story. The farmer was so anxious to have his fields produce a harvest that at night he would go out and pull on the rice stalks to try to make them grow faster! Sometimes we too are tempted to pull on the rice stalks at night in the hopes that they will grow faster but must realize that all we can do is be aware and believe in self and the world. You can be at peace if you have done everything possible to reach your goal in the moment.

You might ask permission and suggest to your client that they experiment with simply sitting and spending ten or fifteen minutes a day doing nothing. If they already practice some form of prayer or meditation that produces a sense of stillness encourage them to use it. What works here is not a reflective self-questioning process, which is intellectual and keeps us psycho-physiologically active. Just have the person be with a simple emptying of the mind.

If the sitting meditation style doesn't work well for your client, encourage them to spend fifteen minutes a day walking alone in silence, while letting thoughts come in and then evaporate. Have them focus on their breathing and their steps. Yoga, Tai Chi, and other quieting practices may be of interest to your client. Support their exploration.

The important thing here is that the quieting practice not be just another thing to do. It needs to be effortless effort. It is a clearing of the mind so that the work done later will be fresher and more focused.

Don't just do something! Sit there!

—Old Zen saying

6. The Welcome Packet. Your client welcome packet (see appendix) should contain powerful, thought-provoking questions well beyond just assembling informational data. Ask your new client what their dreams are! Ask them what they know they must complete in this lifetime to feel fulfilled. Experiment with creating your own welcome packet that is just the right length, not too long and laborious, not too brief and inadequate.

If your client skipped over the more reflective questions in your welcome packet, explore their experience with them. "Tell me about the questions you chose not to answer." You may help them to slow down a minute and realize something about themselves. Are they in just so big of a hurry in life that they felt they couldn't slow down and reflect for a moment? What are they afraid of? Help them find out.

If your client is willing, obtain an agreement to complete the more reflective questions. Explain to them the benefits of doing so for both you and themselves. Set up a good way to hold them accountable for completion.

A Welcome Packet for a more clinical setting might be more brief, but still needs to help the coach see a picture of the client's whole life – work, home and the medical picture. A statement about the clarity of the coaching relationship as related to the client's treatment providers may also be a excellent inclusion.

Laying the Foundation for Coaching

As your coach, it's important for me to understand how you view the world in general, yourself, your family and your job or career. Each person comes from a unique place in their thinking and in the way they interact with the world around them.

Answering these questions clearly and thoughtfully, will serve both you and me. You may find that they help you clarify perceptions about yourself and the direction of your life. These are "pondering" type questions, designed to stimulate your thinking in a way that will make our work together more productive. Take your time answering them. If they are not complete by our first (foundation) session, just bring what you have completed and finish the rest later. These answers will be treated with complete professional confidentiality.

Occupation / nature of business: _____

Employers or Business Name: _____

Date of birth: _____ Marital status_____

Do you have children? _____ Do your children live with you? _____

Coaching

1. What do want to get from the coaching relationship?_____
   _____
   _____

2. What is the "best" way for me to coach you most effectively, what tips would you give to me about what would work best? _____
   _____
   _____

3. Do you have any apprehension or preconceived ideas of coaching? _____
   _____
   _____

Job / Career

1. What do you want from your job / career? _____
   _____
   _____

2. What projects or tasks are you involved in currently or regularly?_____
   _____
   _____

Reproducible Worksheet Masters are available for purchase on CD ROM from Whole Person Associates, 101 W. 2nd St., Suite 203, Duluth, MN 55802, 800-247-6789, www.wholeperson.com.

FIGURE 7.1

Wellness Assessments

Knowing is not enough; we must apply.
Willing is not enough; we must do.

—Johann Wolfgang von Goethe

As we start our lifestyle change journey, a more thorough inventory of our current condition and equipment might be wise. Wellness assessments can help us in ways that our reflective dialogue with our clients does not reach.

Wellness assessments allow us to get more of an actual measurement of where we are to start with, our baseline. Knowing truly where we are, we can measure later to see what progress is made. It's kind of like taking GPS coordinates, or working with our compass to locate where we truly are on the map to start with.

Wellness assessments give our clients feedback on a number of variables that are very relevant and often critical to their health. Wellness assessments often ask questions that would never occur to the client, or even the coach to ask. While more personal questions seem inappropriate early on in a conversation, an inventory can be more forthright.

You would never want to ask your client one hundred questions in one session. However, a wellness assessment can do just that, especially when it is in the convenient form of an online inventory that can be partially completed, cached, and then finished later.

A comprehensive wellness assessment can also be a great learning experience for your client. Some assessments teach as they assess. Clients can increase awareness and gain insight. In addition to feedback, the client also learns what behaviors are associated with good health and which ones with higher risks. Sometimes change can result from the awareness gained from taking the inventory alone.

When we have this baseline information to start with, it is possible to use the assessment instruments again at a later date to chart and measure progress. This is very helpful to the client, and leads to the measurable results we are seeking for them. In situations where an employer is funding the coaching work being done, measurable outcomes (still following rules of confidentiality) are vital.

Simple Wellness Assessments: Tools of Elicitation

Sometimes in finding our way we don't need a highly technical topographic map, we can get started very well with a simple sketch on a piece of paper. The assessment component of wellness coaching is not about pathological diagnosis, it is about increasing awareness. Here we find or create anew, tools that help us elicit from the client, for their own use, information that would not have been discovered otherwise. "Whatever works!" might be the motto here.

The Wheel of Life

A real stand-by of the wellness coach is the Wheel of Life tool. This simple pie-chart approach for rating your own level of satisfaction in eight to nine areas of your life is not to be underestimated. I've been amazed at how startled a person can be once they see how out of balance their life really is when they look at it both graphically and holistically.

The Wheel of Life in Coaching

Rank your level of satisfaction in each area of your life. The closer you are to 10 the more fulfilled you feel. Once you have marked your number in each area, connect each number forming a new outside perimeter for your circle.

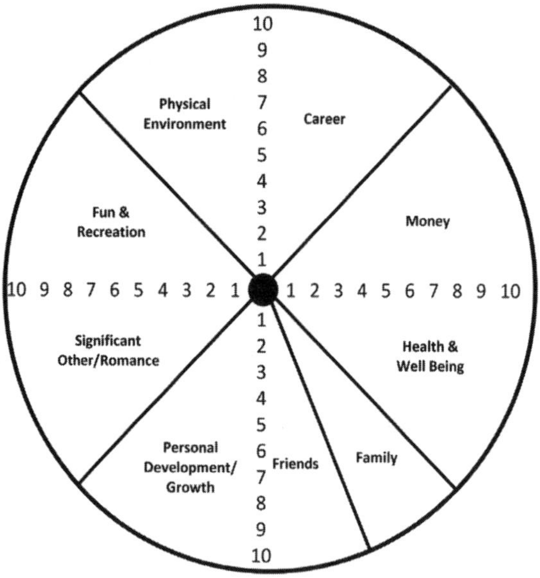

Physical Environment · Career · Fun & Recreation · Money · Significant Other/Romance · Health & Well Being · Personal Development/Growth · Friends · Family

How smooth or bumpy is your life? _____

Are there areas of your life that need attention? _____

What areas of your life are you willing to address now, soon, later? _____

Reproducible Worksheet Masters are available for purchase on CD ROM from Whole Person Associates, 101 W. 2nd St., Suite 203, Duluth, MN 55802, 800-247-6789, www.wholeperson.com.

FIGURE 7.2

Working With The Wheel of Life

Ask your client to mark their level of satisfaction in each dimension of their life. Have them draw a line across each section at their point of satisfaction. Their Wheel of Life should become a circle with a jagged outside edge that reflects the client's satisfaction with their life.

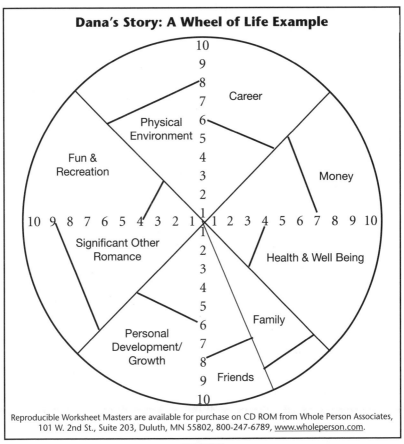

Dana's Story: A Wheel of Life Example

Reproducible Worksheet Masters are available for purchase on CD ROM from Whole Person Associates, 101 W. 2nd St., Suite 203, Duluth, MN 55802, 800-247-6789, www.wholeperson.com.

FIGURE 7.3

Instruct them to reflect on each area. Remind your client that only they define satisfaction. The challenge here is to see the glass half-full, but to not minimize a lack of satisfaction or fulfillment in any area. Reassure them that you will keep their responses entirely confidential.

You can also customize your own wheel of life to cover the eight or nine dimensions of life that you believe are important to living a wellness lifestyle. Here are the nine dimensions that I utilize in the

Wellness Mapping 360° Wheel of Life and the questions you might ask as you coach your client through the results.

Career

1. How fulfilling is your career? Are you content? Is it a good fit for you?

2. On a scale of 1–10 (1 = the least, 10 = the most) how motivated are you to change or develop this aspect of your life?

3. If you are up for some improvement, what is one small action you can take this week to either find out more about changing in this area, or to actually make a small behavioral change?

Money

1. Describe the stress (if any) that you experience around the issue of money. Describe your "relationship" with money (stable, unpredictable, volatile, rewarding, frustrating, etc.) . . . elaborate.

2. On a scale of 1–10 (1 = the least, 10 = the most) how motivated are you to change or develop this aspect of your life?

3. If you are up for some improvement, what is one small action you can take this week to either find out more about changing in this area, or to actually make a small behavioral change?

Health/Wellbeing

1. Describe any health challenges that you currently face. Describe any particular joys you experience about your health. Describe the level of health you want to experience five years from now.

2. On a scale of 1–10 (1 = the least, 10 = the most) how motivated are you to change or develop this aspect of your life?

3. If you are up for some improvement, what is one small action you can take this week to either find out more about changing in this area, or to actually make a small behavioral change?

Family Relationships

1. How fulfilling is your relationship with your own

immediate family and/or your family of origin? How satisfied are you with the level of closeness and support that you feel between yourself and others in the family. Are you able to get many of your needs met through your family?

2. On a scale of 1–10 (1 = the least, 10 = the most) how motivated are you to change or develop this aspect of your life?

3. If you are up for some improvement, what is one small action you can take this week to either find out more about changing in this area, or to actually make a small behavioral change?

Friends

1. Friendship is about both quality and quantity. Do you have enough friends, and close enough friends to meet your needs? Have you created any new friendships in the last two years?

2. On a scale of 1–10 (1 = the least, 10 = the most) how motivated are you to change or develop this aspect of your life?

3. If you are up for some improvement, what is one small action you can take this week to either find out more about changing in this area, or to actually make a small behavioral change?

Personal Growth/Development

1. Do you invest enough time, energy and money in your own personal growth and development, including spiritual development?

2. On a scale of 1–10 (1 = the least, 10 = the most) how motivated are you to change or develop this aspect of your life?

3. If you are up for some improvement, what is one small action you can take this week to either find out more about changing in this area, or to actually make a small behavioral change?

Significant Other/Romance

1. Are you at peace with this aspect of your life? If this is still an active part of your life, are your needs getting met well in this area?

2. On a scale of 1–10 (1 = the least, 10 = the most) how motivated are you to change or develop this aspect of your life?

3. If you are up for some improvement, what is one small action you can take this week to either find out more about changing in this area, or to actually make a small behavioral change?

Fun & Recreation

1. Do you invest enough time, energy and money, in having fun and re-creating yourself? Do you allow yourself to adequately value this way of re-energizing and re-vitalizing yourself?

2. On a scale of 1–10 (1 = the least, 10 = the most) how motivated are you to change or develop this aspect of your life?

3. If you are up for some improvement, what is one small action you can take this week to either find out more about changing in this area, or to actually make a small behavioral change?

Environment

1. How satisfied are you with the home, neighborhood, workplace, and surrounding landscape/environment where you live? Does is contribute well to your quality of life, or challenge it?

2. On a scale of 1–10 (1 = the least, 10 = the most) how motivated are you to change or develop this aspect of your life?

3. If you are up for some improvement, what is one small action you can take this week to either find out more about changing in this area, or to actually make a small behavioral change?

Balance and Fulfillment for Your Client

As you go over the completed wheel of life with your client, you will be helping them see how balanced and fulfilling their lives are. The level of satisfaction in each area (1-10) is their level of fulfillment in that area. The relationship between all of the dimensions and levels of satisfaction displays the reality of balance in their lives. Ask them to answer the question "How well does your wheel roll?"

As we said earlier, suggest to your client that they look at their wheel in the following way. Instead of imagining that this pie chart is a wheel with the outer rim being the pie chart outer circle, have them imagine that the rim of the wheel is really the "rim" they have drawn with their combined satisfaction ratings. Most people find that their ride is not as smooth as they thought or desire! A high rating in several areas and low ratings in others makes the wheel go "ka-womp, ka-womp" down the street of life.

The Pie-Chart Advantage

You could ask your client to list their rating of satisfaction on several dimensions of wellness/life in a vertical list. While you both would probably gain some valuable information to work with, you would lose a couple of distinct advantages the circle offers.

The circular pie chart helps the client see each dimension equally. Vertical lists inevitably engender a rank-ordering of their content, implying that number one is more important than number two, etc. The pie-chart allows the client to assign his or her own level of value to each area.

COACHING NOTE

The reason the Wheel of Life I use has nine dimensions instead of the eight that would maintain a nice symmetry is worth noting. In other wheel of life tools I've seen, the dimensions of family and friends are often combined. As I worked with clients this combination of friends & family often puzzled them. Frequently I got ratings in the 4-6 range. When I would enquire about this I often got responses like "Well, my friends are awesome, a ten, and my family is awful, a zero, so that's a five, right?" When I broke the nice symmetry of the chart and separated out these two areas I got the real story. I found this especially valuable because understanding the client's support system (and lack thereof) is critical in helping them make lasting lifestyle change. So—nine dimensions. It works.

The wheel approach uses the power of a strong visual graphic to engage different parts of the brain and help the client see relationships between dimensions. You may be able to effectively engage your client in an exploration of how their career satisfaction is indeed related to the level of satisfaction they experience in family, money, fun and recreation.

Uses of The Wheel of Life

The Wheel of Life is a great tool to include in a client welcome packet. It can allow you to have a solid starting place in your foundation session. Before launching into each dimension I always ask the client to tell me about their experience in completing the wheel. What was it like? How did they feel during and after completing it? What did they realize or become aware of by completing it?

You can also use the Wheel of Life in other settings such as workshops, or even at booths at health expos. It's a quick and easy tool to complete and can stimulate curiosity about one's wellness. I even had one client begin coaching with me after he approached me following a workshop with his Wheel of Life of in hand and merely stated "My wheel won't roll!"

The Wheel of Life is a great health promotion and education tool. What I like about it is that it really points your services (or that of your program's) in the direction of individualizing wellness. It shows your client (or employees) that their own evaluation of satisfaction in these areas is quite valid as an important aspect of their health and wellbeing. Yes, blood pressure numbers are important, but so is satisfaction with one's life.

Make Your Own Wheel of Life

Try adapting this pie format to the particular focus that your coaching client might need. Perhaps you have a client who is focusing on physical fitness. A quick snapshot of their satisfaction in this area can be obtained, with more accuracy and detail, by using a Wheel of Life modified for this purpose.

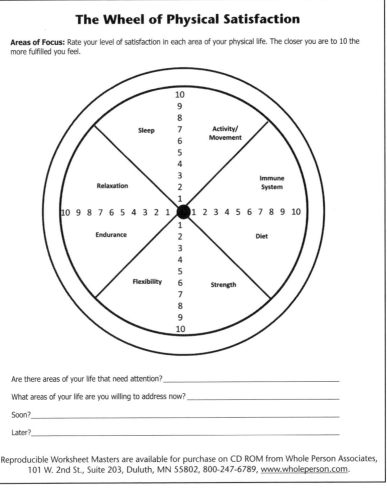

The Wheel of Physical Satisfaction

Areas of Focus: Rate your level of satisfaction in each area of your physical life. The closer you are to 10 the more fulfilled you feel.

Are there areas of your life that need attention? _____

What areas of your life are you willing to address now? _____

Soon?_____

Later?_____

Reproducible Worksheet Masters are available for purchase on CD ROM from Whole Person Associates, 101 W. 2nd St., Suite 203, Duluth, MN 55802, 800-247-6789, www.wholeperson.com.

FIGURE 7.4

By working with this wheel (Figure 7.4) we help our client see that physical fitness, and their satisfaction with it, is not a simple all-or-nothing concept. When asking a client how satisfied are they with their general physical fitness you may trigger a different story in every person. For some clients the question will translate into "So! Just how fat are you?," and all the self-judgment that is carried with that question. Looking at physical fitness from an eight dimensional perspective (as in the wheel above) gives the client the message that there is more to physical fitness than just strength, or waistline measurements.

It also allows the client and coach to see ways to co-create a wellness plan that will really get at the specific areas where there is the least satisfaction.

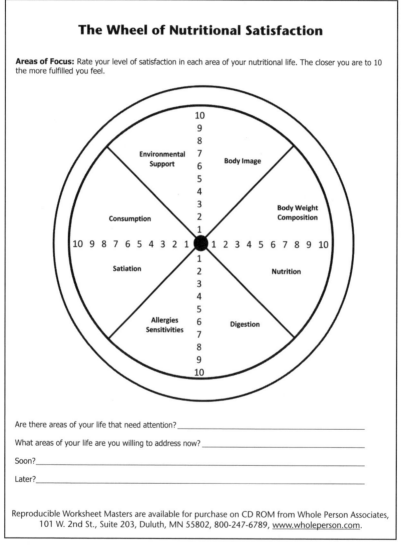

FIGURE 7.5

Formal Wellness Assessments

HRAs

Wellness programs found in corporations, hospitals, fitness centers, etc.are often built around the most basic of wellness assessments, the Health Risk Assessment, or HRA. Developed early in the wellness movement, HRAs are still in widespread use today. Over 50 HRAs are on the market aiming to help individuals and organizations reduce health risks by identifying the correlations between behavior and health for each individual.

The idea is to increase awareness in the participant of the lifestyle behaviors they perform that increase their risk of illness and premature death. Due to years of research, it is now easy for us to conclude that the more someone smokes tobacco, the greater the health risk they experience. It's all probabilities, but the message is clear: behave in these ways and you increase your risks and may not live as long; behave in these other ways and you decrease your risks and may even live longer. HRAs have become more sophisticated than the early models that pioneered the field. They look at more than just smoking, drinking, and seat belt usage. Many of the risk factors are associated with coronary heart disease and cancer. Some HRAs include the risks of unsafe sex being practiced in the age of HIV/AIDS. Some look at the more psychological side of health.

HRAs are used primarily as feedback devices for the people who take them. The key to their effectiveness is the nature and quality of that feedback. Increasingly online-based, HRAs are often providing extensive links to support resources that provide the client with tons of health information and even tools for tracking their own lifestyle change attempts. Better HRAs have built into them some form of change readiness scale (e.g. Prochaska, et.al.), or if not, change readiness may be assessed in feedback sessions through direct questioning.

One of the most common scenarios is for a company to incentivize their employees to take an HRA, usually online. Paper and pencil HRAs are available too and are machine scored. The employee/client is then given feedback in a number of ways that range from low to higher effectiveness.

1. The client may simply be mailed the results, or be able to see them online with instructions written as to what the results mean.

2. The client is set up with a telephone appointment with someone who spends 15-20 minutes on the phone going over the results with the employee. The test interpretor may have training that ranges from minimal to very good. In a good system these people are typically some type of health specialist, such as LPNs, fitness specialists, or trained health coaches.

3. Another step up is when HRAs are combined with the gathering of biometric data (actual measurements such as blood pressure, blood work results, BMI, etc.) taken by health specialists, and then either a telephone or, better still, live appointment, is made to review and interpret the results and answer questions.

4. If the program is fairly comprehensive and woven into the larger employee health benefits resources, the assessment may result in a referral to an Employee Assistance Program (EAP), an employee's clinic, a physician, etc. Here, an employee may get valuable help or medical intervention for a condition that was going undiagnosed and untreated.

5. In the best programs, at least a taste of what we might call more complete wellness coaching takes place. If the educator interpreting the results is a trained wellness coach, the results may go to a different level. Even in a system where time is severely limited, the coach approach may allow the client to build some trust with the wellness coach, and determine a direction of focus. After a brief exploration with the coach listening on a professional level, the coach helps the client leave with a sense of ownership of their health, what they want to work on, and a system of accountability regarding it.

6. The system may opt for some participants (perhaps especially those at high risk) to have follow-up coaching sessions based on the results. Even brief (ten-minute) follow-up phone calls every quarter and regular e-mails can have some effectiveness.

The Down Side of HRAs

Some critics of Health Risk Assessments point out that there are disadvantages to HRA usage. When the first bit of feedback you receive about your health is what age you are predicted to die, it may be hard to hear! Not all HRAs hit you with this message first, but a criticism of HRAs is that they can tend to paint a picture of morbidity and the postponement of the inevitable. While some see this as merely a dose of reality therapy for us all, others would argue that it is a poor motivator. Do we change our health behavior out of fear alone? Can we be scared straight into buckling that seat belt, and eating our high-fiber vegetables?

One would think that an employee required to take an HRA would be happy that they are getting a free health assessment that is designed to help them be healthy and recognize ways to improve their health. However, in an organization where trust is an issue, and where there is fear that one's job may be in jeopardy if one's health is anything but excellent, how honest will answers be? How reliable is the HRA if an employee is telling management what they want to hear?

Coaching With HRAs

Health Risk Assessments are often the gateway through which clients come to the wellness coach within an organization whose wellness program is centered on reducing health risks. Employees are often incentivized (often with surprisingly large amounts of cash) to complete the HRA. Individuals with multiple health risks and/or chronic illnesses are then invited to make use of the available wellness coaching.

A challenge for the wellness coach working with a client who has just taken an HRA is to maintain the wellness coaching mindset of advocate and inspire. The temptation with the diagnostic nature of the HRA is to shift into the diagnose and treat model and start prescribing to the client instead of remaining their ally. Instruments that point out the client's risky behaviors may come across as judgments about the behavior. It is easy for some clients to feel like they are wrong and not OK. The coach's task is to be aware of this possibility and help the client see that the instrument is not so personal. Certain behaviors are statistically correlated with increased incidence of illness, injury and other negative results, and it's recommended that you behave this other way instead, and that's all that is being said.

For many wellness coaches the HRA is a standard tool that is part of the system they work in. For the solo wellness coach, who is in business for themselves, the HRA is another instrument to consider and to know how to use. You may find that you like to have it as an option, and discover that with certain clients it really provides something that they are looking for, and something that will fit in with what motivates them to change.

Dee Edington, on of the pioneers of the HRA while leading The University of Michigan Health Management Research Center, provides us with a new look at the value of both HRA's and coaching. Dr. Edington, in his recent book *Zero Trends: Health As A Serious Economic Strategy*, states that an effective wellness program need three elements: a good HRA, biometric screening, and health/wellness coaching. He argues that reserving coaching just for the high risk individuals ignores the fact that the low risk population, if ignored, will "migrate" into the high risk columns by developing more and more health risks over time. "Keeping the healthy people healthy" may be the most effective, and in the long run, economical approach to wellness.

"Everyone can use a health coach."

Dee Edington

The Wellness Inventory

The Wellness Inventory (WI) was the first true wellness assessment instrument created. It was developed initially in 1976 by John W. Travis, M.D. Jim Strohecker through HealthWorld Online (www.my-wellnesstest.com) developed the extensive online delivery system it is today.

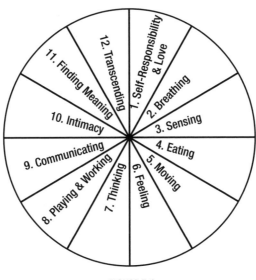

FIGURE 7.6

The WI conceives of wellness in a 12-dimensional model (wellness energy system) that gives an inclusive and unique view of what healthy wellness lifestyles include.

1. Self-Responsibility and Love
2. Breathing (and relaxing)
3. Sensing
4. Eating
5. Moving
6. Feeling
7. Thinking
8. Playing and Working
9. Communicating
10. Intimacy and Sex
11. Finding Meaning
12. Transcending

In *The Wellness Workbook* (Travis & Ryan), Travis elaborates on each of these dimensions. For the wellness coach there are some immediate advantages to this unusual way of looking at wellness. Instead of confronting your client with the topic of exercise, which I find many clients to be almost phobic about, you can talk about movement in their lives. Instead of diet, you speak about eating and it can open up a broader exploration of the role that eating and food plays in their life.

The inclusion of dimensions such as feeling, thinking, communicating and intimacy & sex opens up the more mental/emotional sides of wellness and reinforces that wellness is much more than just diet and exercise. The dimensions of finding meaning and transcendence open up the philosophical and the spiritual areas for exploration. Using Travis's energy model you can see how self-responsibility & love provides the foundation for a wellness, breathing, sensing and eating are our primary ways of taking in energy, and the remaining eight dimensions are ways we output energy.

Taking the WI is a very self-educative wellness experience. All the questions are stated in positive statement terms. An example is "I recognize that responsibility for my health lies within me, rather than with an outside authority." The client then answers each item by indicating how true it is for them (Yes/Always/Usually, Often, Sometimes/Maybe, Occasionally, or No/Never/Hardly Ever). They are then immediately asked how satisfied they are with their response. The content of the items themselves is a tutorial on factors involved in living a wellness lifestyle. Your client can also click on any topic and find a complete description of it, and can also access further resources and information on each area in the resource section.

The WI is actually set up online as a one-year wellness and lifestyle change program.

Step 1—Assessment: Complete a whole person assessment in the 12 dimensions of wellness and lifestyle.

Step 2—Scores: Receive Wellness & Satisfaction Scores in each section. Discover where you are most motivated to change.

Step 3—Personal Wellness Plan: Create 3-5 wellness action steps in the areas you are most motivated to change.

Step 4—Tools to Help You Reach Your Goals: Utilize tools to help you follow your wellness plan and meet your goals.

Step 5—Supporting Ongoing Wellness: Re-assess in six months and monitor your progress. Optional wellness coaching.

Common to online inventories, the administrator (in this case the coach) has confidentially protected access to scores so they can review the WI results with their client, even telephonically by looking at the same online screens at the same time.

The Wellness Inventory now features two scores. One is your "wellness score" which shows how close to the optimal wellness response the client has indicated their behavior is. The second is a valuable Readiness For Change score where the client has been asked to rate how ready they are (1-10 scale) to take action on changing that behavior in the next six months. This is a vast improvement over the inventory's old "satisfaction score", and will be very useful for the coach and client to work on together.

You might have your client complete the built-in wellness planning process and go over it together with them. Ask them in detail about it and look for ways to strategize with them to make it operational and build in the accountability they desire regarding their plan.

The WI has a fairly sophisticated vocabulary and explores more psychological and philosophical concepts. Many coaches find that clients need a minimum of a high school education.

Physiological Measures

One concrete advantage that wellness coaching enjoys is that some of its more important outcomes are quite measurable. While we can probably never really pinpoint the variable(s) responsible for a shift in the physiological functioning of our client, we can often look for physical changes that can be measured. A decrease in blood pressure, an improvement in blood-work measures, an increase in endurance, a reduction in percentage of body fat, more hours of restful sleep, are all benchmarks that progress is being made.

The realm of taking some of the more sophisticated physiological measures falls into the world of treatment where the coach becomes an ally to the healthcare specialist. Anyone can step on the scale, move the notch on the belt, or time their assent of a steep nearby hill, but the professional work of coaching lies somewhere between simple self-observations and the more medically oriented work.

Let the nurse practitioner take your client's blood pressure. Work with your client's M.D. and the treatment program they have prescribed. Be a coach about it. Work as your client's coach and not their healthcare provider. Stick with your effective and vital role of helping your client with the behavioral aspects of medical compliance. Help your client actually do what their treatment program directs them to do with their lifestyle.

Combining wellness inventories and/or HRAs with actual physiological measurements, or biometric data, is a powerful method. It gives your client an accurate picture of where they are. When their LDL cholesterol score is compared with the healthier range that is expected, they know what they need to shoot for. You are there to help them with the lifestyle component of making that happen.

One of the most common physiological goals is to attain a healthy weight. A few words here are important. In working with individuals seeking a healthier weight, a common error is to look solely at pounds/kilos lost. It is misleading because when your client begins to exercise, they are increasing muscle mass. This is good, but muscle weighs more than fat! The Body Mass Index, or BMI, is an approximation based upon finding your height and weight on a chart and seeing how you stack up. Differences in body type are not factored in well, nor are health conditions that affect overall height (such as scoliosis, etc.). While the BMI has contributed greatly to research, the wellness coach has to use it with caution.

Percent body fat is often held by exercise physiologists to be the single best measurement to take to show healthy body composition change. Have your client get a good measurement from a personal fitness trainer, an exercise physiologist, or someone trained in the how to of this process. There are now at least four different ways to ascertain percentage of body fat.

Because fat floats taking body weight under water is probably the most accurate measurement! Some health clubs have monthly hydrostatic weigh-ins at their swimming pools. There are electronic devices on the market now that resemble a simple set of bathroom scales, but electrically measure bio impedance through the body and calculate percent body fat that way.

A much more convenient method is the simple circumference measuring methods like the one developed by the U.S. Navy, however this seems to fall victim to all the problems that the BMI does. Much more accurate and almost as easy to do are the skin-fold caliper measurements. When taken by a trained specialist, the Academy of Sports

Medicine says these methods are 98% accurate. The central challenge with results of any assessment you work with is helping your client to determine what their goals should be. What is the ideal percentage of body fat for them? Perhaps a better question is "What is the most healthy body composition for me?" Individual factors abound. Is your client a sedentary couch potato, a competitive weight lifter or a long-distance runner?

The effective wellness coach helps their client work with physical measurements, but helps them put it all in the context of their over-all health and wellness goals. The measurements can provide helpful benchmarks of progress, or reminders of extra effort required along the way. Ask your client what will work as the best feedback for them. It's all part of co-creating the wellness plan in our next chapter.

Coach First, Measure Second

A word to the wise . . . If you are like many health educators, who typically begin an initial session with a client by taking physical measurements such as weight, height, waist circumference, etc., you might consider not taking any measurements at the first contact. While your client may expect this, give them the unexpected! Talk to them. Coach them with great listening. Hear their story. Coach them with powerful questions that help them to explore what their weight issue means to them. Explore all their tried and failed experiences. Ask how they hope this one will be different.

When we take biometric data upon first contact it can feel like we are judging the person. It may feel like we are evaluating what is wrong with them. It can put them through a process that reminds them of numerous times in the past where they have felt ashamed. In the coach mindset, as opposed to the medical mindset, we are here to form an alliance for change with them, not to provide treatment. Set the tone by being their coach first!

> *There is a human striving for self-transcendence. It's part of what makes us human. With all of our flaws we want to go a little bit further than we've gone before and maybe even further than anyone else has gone before.*
>
> —George B. Leonard

Chapter 8

Charting the Course of Change: Wellness Mapping 360°™ Part II

Human life is a journey whose end is not in sight.
Searching, longing and questioning is in our DNA. Who we
are and what we will become is determined by the questions
that animate us, and by those we refuse to ask. Your
questions are your quest. As you ask, so shall you be.

—**Sam Keen**

The Personal Map or Plan

You've assisted your wellness coaching client to take stock of their life and identify where they want to go. Together you've set a firm foundation place to start from and helped them to see what some of their strengths and challenges are. You've established an alliance with them so they know they don't have to take this journey alone. Now is the time to create the map.

Co-creating the Wellness Plan

To insure commitment and motivation, let the development of a wellness plan be a process of co-creation that gives your client a clear map to follow. Stay in the coach mindset of advocate and inspire. It may seem so absolutely obvious that your client needs _____! In reality, if your client did in fact do blank, everything might work out just fine. The prescribe-and treat-approach may seductively appear to be much more time efficient. You might think that you could just write up a great plan for your client, like a prescription, and expect that they would thankfully take it and implement it. Your client may even be pleading for you to "Just tell me what to do!" Your challenge, as a coach, especially if you have a healthcare background, is not to create a treatment plan.

One of the real advantages of wellness coaching is that it is different than what your client has tried before. Wellness coaching is different because the client takes responsibility for their own health and wellness and because they improve their lives themselves. Chances are great that your client will have already been there and done that with prescriptive approaches. They've had books, talk-show celebrities on TV, healthcare professionals, gym teachers, friends, parents and others recommend, cajole, intimidate, frighten, shame, manipulate and lovingly urge them to change by telling them what to do. Yet here they are, still stuck.

All these other people have stood at the bottom of the mountain and told the person how to climb it. They've recommended a route, told them what equipment to carry, patted them on the back and wished them well. The wellness coach goes up on the mountain with their client. The coach doesn't climb the mountain for the client, they serve as a guide for them.

You can offer a framework for creating a wellness map to help your client get started. They will be the one completing the framework, filling in the blanks. Your coaching skills can come forth and help them with strategizing, prioritizing, challenging, encouraging and acknowledging. You can help the person to dis-invite their inner critic or gremlin from participating in the creation of their plan. That same gremlin loves to discourage the person or build in self-defeating components to keep them from changing and instead cling to the comfort of the *status quo*. Help them identify gremlin talk and keep it out of the wellness plan.

Make your approach to wellness planning growth oriented. Instead of a wellness plan consider calling it a wellness growth plan. When your client sees the connection between being well and his or her own personal growth, motivation will be even stronger. Actualizing potential in all dimensions of a person's life as defined by that person, is the ultimate wellness process.

Drawing The Map—The Essential Components of the Wellness Plan

When you look at many general wellness plans you often find various prescriptive formulas for being healthy and well. Eat this, exercise this way, get more sleep, etc. In wellness coaching, the customized wellness plan is really a map or a tool that helps your client to:

- Find their way by identifying specifically how they want to work on improving their lifestyle

- Set up ways to measure and track progress

- Secure adequate support

- Identify outcomes so they know when they have arrived at their destination.

From the world of coaching we may discover various action plans. Some of these models may work fine with wellness coaching, however we need to be careful not to emphasize an action-only approach. Motivation, blocks to completion, support resources all deserve consideration as well. Wellness coaching is about lifestyle improvement – lifestyle change and maintaining that positive change. The wellness growth plan looks at the questions of "How can I grow further, and actualize more of my potential?" "How can I improve myself in these ways?"

Wellness plans can be very simple, even focused on one area at a time. On the other extreme they can become so complex and inclusive that they become cumbersome and are often totally abandoned. Your coaching challenge is to work with your client to strike a balance that is effective and suits them best. We do know that success promotes success. For some clients the baby steps approach works best; others are ready to make huge strides!

Here is the Wellness Mapping 360°™ Methodology for co-creating the wellness plan: the Wellness Map. We begin by helping our clients craft a vision.

The Well-Life Vision

Your client's keen and thorough awareness of where they are at becomes the starting place for our journey, but how clear are we on where we are going? As we showed in an earlier chapter, a clear idea of what we desire can be a powerful motivator that pulls us forward.

Think of a buried treasure map, like in a pirate movie. There is always the "You are here" spot on the map and then that coveted "X" where the treasure is hidden. If "X marks the spot" then we need to place it on our map that we are creating for this wellness journey.

A client of mine needed and wanted to lose one hundred pounds. She was a single mother with two young daughters and it broke her heart that she could not share with them something that she loved. Growing up at the foot of the Rocky Mountains, she had been hiking and camping in those mountains since childhood and now it was just a dear, but distant memory. She wanted so much to share that way of growing up with her girls. We coached together and what powerfully motivated her to implement her Wellness Plan was the Well-Life Vision she created.

All day long at her sedentary job she found ways to increase her movement, and measured all her movement with an activity-monitoring device. She meal-planned and tracked calories with her phone-app. At the end of the day when she came home tired and the device on her belt told her that her movement goal for the day was short, she faced what we all usually face at that moment: sit or move, accept a lack of progress, or keep making it. That was when she would remember her Well-Life Vision: a crystal clear picture in her mind of walking in the mountains down a beautiful forested trail with sunlight beaming through the aspen trees as her two daughters ran ahead laughing. This was the tipping point that she needed. She kicked off her work shoes, put on her walking shoes, and went out for two more miles (again, and again).

I'm happy to say that this client maintained her motivation, lost her first forty pounds while we were working together and begin to be able to finally get back into those mountains with her little girls.

A Well-Life Vision is not just a day-dream, a fantasy. We want it to be an image that represents the way we want to live when we are living our best life possible. It is *who we want to be*, not just what we are doing. Living that way allows us to be that relaxed, caring and generous self, instead of that anxious, worried, or lethargic person we've become. It epitomizes our values. We see ourselves living in a way that is in complete accordance with our values and our priorities.

For that image to work for us we need it to be something we believe may be a "stretch", but it is obtainable, and obtainable not so far into the future. We aren't talking about retirement plans here, we're talking about seeing how by making certain changes in our lifestyle we could actually create a better way of living in the near future. "If I make these changes, if I do *this* right now, it's a step towards living the way I really want to live." So, going on our half-hour walk at noon feels like a step that is connected to that picture we have of ourselves out on the dance floor moving fluidly among our good friends.

Creating a Well-Life Vision

While we constantly coach through a process of co-creation, the Well-Life Vision is truly our client's own creation. We "co-create" by helping them with the process, and perhaps with a tool like The Well-Life Vision Tool (see Tool Kit).

Create a List

Creating the Well-Life Vision usually starts with a coaching conversation that generates a list of qualities the client would like to see in that best-life-possible of theirs: healthy relationships with co-workers, intimate partners, family, and friends; a healthy body able to move effortlessly and vigorously, a sense of meaning and purpose, being tobacco-free, being able to enjoy sports or activities that they love, etc.

The coaching process sometimes delves into values clarification, prioritization of what is really important to that person, even meaning and purpose in life. It's all good. The wisdom in life is in the journey, not just in reaching a destination.

Develop a Statement

From that rambling list we want to help our clients synthesize a crisp, motivating statement that captures what they are talking about. From two or three paragraphs, we help them reduce it to one or two sentences.

My Well-Life Vision is to be healthy and well enough as I age to be able to share the outdoors with my grandchildren like I did with my children.

Now, for me to be able to live that Well-Life Vision, what does it mean I have to do on a regular basis? It may mean that I have to be able to hike, camp, canoe, and travel easily and that requires a certain level of health and physical fitness. So from a crystal clear image in my mind of me hiking along a creek with my grandchildren, playing with them as they wade in the shallows and look for minnows and crayfish, we go to the implication that in order to be able to do that, I need to go ahead and take a mid-day break and go for that half-hour walk, and later on go out to dinner and restrain myself from ordering the French fries. The implication is that in order to live my Well-Life Vision I have to be actively living my Wellness Plan.

Create an Image

The Well-Life Vision Statement may be all your client needs, but if they are good at visualization, then take advantage of this powerful additional process. For some clients creating detailed images in their minds is tough work, for others an IMAX movie screen is right there inside of their craniums. Have your client take all their thoughts about their Well-Life vision, perhaps with you helping by summarizing what you've heard, and urge them to imagine that they are a movie producer capable of creating any scene possible that could represent their vision. Urge them to think in symbolic or metaphorical ways. If they are more concrete about it that can be fine too.

A good image of your client's vision is one where in order to be "in" that scene they will have had to accomplish living much of their Wellness Plan. In order for me to see myself hiking with my grandchildren and see myself moving so easily, I have to be at a certain level of physical fitness. In order to be there with them I have to be managing my work/life balance well enough to have that free time with them. The motivational link is there and connected to a picture of real joy.

Every client will come up with their own style of Well-Life Vision. Some will be incredibly creative, symbolic and intriguing. Others will simply describe a vision of simple contentment. Contentment is often highly underrated! Sometime your client will come up with a Well-Life Vision that is very puzzling to you, but at some level it will make sense to them.

I had been working with a middle-aged client who was overweight, a smoker, and had recently had a stroke. Her job was very demanding and often prevented her from exercising and eating the way she want-ed to. She enjoyed big-city living very much and had a good support system. Progress was slow as we explored her whole life and began supporting her on working in more movement and healthier eating. When we coached on developing her Well-Life Vision she came up with a scene that she was very pleased with, but which puzzled me. In her Well-Life Vision she saw herself leaving work early on a week day, going to an outdoor café to meet a girlfriend and seeing the two of them sitting in the sunshine, sipping a "skinny latte'" and laughing. That was it.

I struggled to see how this related to the health goals she had been working on, but finally after a breakthrough coaching session I saw the connection. The essence of her vision was that she wanted to be managing the stress of her job so well that she could take off early on a weekday, meet a friend, sit in the sunshine and laugh! Coaching about her work stress yielded the traction she needed to break through her barriers and make progress on weight loss. After a holiday break she showed up at her appointment announcing she had been tobacco-free for two months, and we hadn't even included working that in her Wellness Plan.

Make sure you and your client have taken the time to forge the coaching alliance and helped them do adequate exploration before you launch into creating a Well-Life Vision. Get to know your client first. Build the coaching relationship so your client trusts you with their hopes and dreams.

Coaching to the Gap

A classic part of Life Coaching is a concept called "coaching to the gap." It's simply the gap between where you are and where you want to be. The powerful question is: "What has to change for you to get there?" A business coach might work with an entrepreneurial client whose business is struggling and unprofitable. They explore all as-pects of the current business practices and the client's interpersonal customer and management style. They get a clear vision of the profit-able and meaningful business that the client wants. They then engage in the process of identifying what has to change about the client them-selves, and their way of doing business for that vision to be realized.

You may begin working with a wellness coaching client who is poorly managing a chronic health condition. Their diet has not changed much since they were diagnosed even though that is essential. They have remained largely sedentary. They get a medical update on their health status and coach with you to explore their whole life and develop a fantastic Well-Life Vision.

They want to live a life that is healthy and well, where movement is easy and their energy level at work is good. They want to be able to travel easily and see the world.

So, we have our client take a deep breath and ask themselves "What needs to change for me to achieve my Well-Life Vision?" Your client explores this question with you in coaching and concludes that they need to focus on improving their medical compliance/adherence, attaining and maintaining a healthy weight, and change their way of dealing with stress in their life. Now we have Areas of Focus to begin creating our map.

Coaching to the Gap

Where I am now -> ----------------> Where I want to be
(Current health status)   (Well Life Vision)

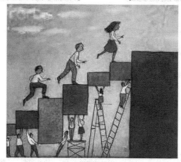

What has to change in my life for me to bridge the gap - to attain my Well Life Vision?

What has to change in your life (and you are ready to change) becomes the areas you focus on.

FIGURE 8.1

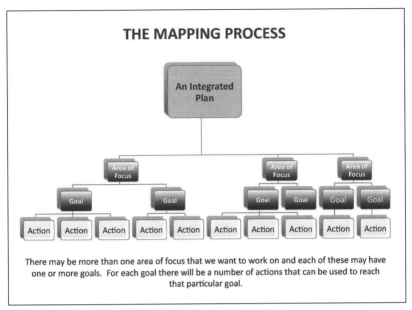

FIGURE 8.2

"Well" Beyond Goal Setting – An Integrated Plan

All too often wellness coaches are trained to simply help clients get clear about setting "health goals" and then taught to provide accountability and support to help their clients succeed. While not bad, we can do so much better.

As seen in the graphic above there is a natural flow to the distinctions made between Areas of Focus, Goals and Action Steps. This taxonomy is not just semantic. The flow we want is a motivational flow. From Action Step to Areas of Focus, your client sees the connection; they have a "reason" to take action. So for the client who has determined that one Area of Focus is to attain and maintain a healthy weight, one Goal is to increase activity (another might be to improve nutrition and eating behavior). To help them achieve that Goal of increased activity the client commits to the Action Step this week of walking at least three times for thirty minutes each time. When out on the walk they realize "why" they are doing it.

All too often coaches focus only on the Action Steps and call them goals. "What are your goals for this week?" In our example the act of walking is not a goal in and of itself. Instead it is a committed action that helps the client achieve their goal.

Here is an example of a Wellness Mapping 360°™ Wellness Map that a client challenged with diabetes might create.

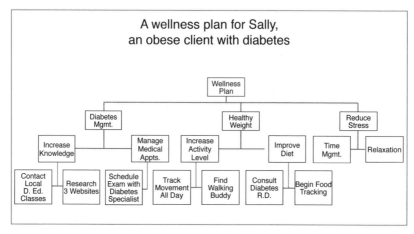

FIGURE 8.3

What to Work On: Areas of Focus

Help your client to be specific. Perhaps draw upon what they learned in completing a tool like the Wellness Wheel to help them identify areas that they want to work on and improve. This becomes the beginning of their Wellness Plan.

For maximum success, prioritize no more than five areas, preferably three to four, and make those areas the ones where there is the greatest readiness for change. Lifestyle prescriptions from healthcare providers and results/feedback from wellness assessment instruments can also factor into the prioritizing process.

Goals: A New Look

A key part of our Integrated Plan is helping our clients determine the goals that will help them experience success in each Area of Focus. We've been careful not to take on too many Areas of Focus, now we have to be strategic and smart when it comes to how many goals to design into each Area of Focus. When coaches confuse Action Steps with Goals there can be a lot of them! Clients who get excited about improving their lifestyles sometimes push for a "total make-over", yet taking on too much and falling short or failing all together is a classic self-defeating pattern for many.

As we saw in determining Areas of Focus, this again is where Readiness For Change Theory comes in and serves us very well. (As we will see later in this chapter.) Your client may be quite ready to modify their diet and way of eating, but not at all ready to begin a conscious exercise program. We want our clients to experience success, especially as they start their wellness journey. Help them select goals with the highest levels of readiness where the probability of success is greater. Let their success build confidence in themselves, the coaching process and in you their coach!

Action Steps: Getting Things Done

If we were to imagine our Integrated Wellness Plan (as shown in the graphic) being like the root system of a giant tree, the taproot would drop down and split into the major roots (our Areas of Focus) and then into the roots that support those major roots (our Goals). The way that trees absorb their water and nourishment from the soil is through the root-hairs at the end of each root. Here where the action is are our Action Steps. Great ideas come down to moving our feet. As the saying goes "You've got to put legs under it." Does it mater how much you love someone if you don't express it?

At each coaching session client and coach co-create Action Steps that the client sees the value in committing to. The best Action Steps are ones where the client sees the motivational link between what they want to achieve and how this concrete step will help them get there. These Action Steps change as progress is made or as challenges demand a different strategy.

A critical part of setting Action Steps is helping our clients answer the question "How will you know when you are being successful?" This is where we have to set criteria for success, or what we might call Indicators of Success. For example: a client may have determined that an Area of Focus for them is improved energy. They are chronically sleep-deprived and set a goal of achieving adequate sleep. But what does "adequate" sleep mean, and how are they going to experiment at getting it? Under the Goal of Getting More Sleep they commit to getting to bed at an earlier hour.

Through our coaching process the client realizes that they need to get clear about what time they will go to bed by (say 10:00 pm on a work night) and how many times a week of achieving this criterion would be satisfactory (at least four nights a week). Now the client has something concrete to shoot for. The indicator of success is set and we can coach the client towards hitting their target. It may sound a bit compulsive here, but this is where real behavioral change often takes place.

For each Area of Focus:

- **Desires:** What do you want?
  In the client's own words, what are the stated desires for this area of focus? This is good to state as both an immediate goal (e.g. lose ten pounds) and a longer-term, more motivational goal (e.g. I want to climb a 14,000 foot/4,267meter peak this summer).

- **Current Location:** Where are you currently?
  Current status of the area of focus the client wants to work on. For example, current percent body fat; hours of sleep/night; 1–10 scale self-ratings of situations or levels of conditioning, etc.

- **Destination:** Where do you want to go? Who do you want to become?
  What that will look like, stated specifically and as measurably as possible.

- **Committed Course:** What are you, the client, making a commitment to do?
  The action steps involved, stated very specifically. Through coaching the client arrives at success-insuring action strategies that are challenging yet attainable.

- **Challenges:** What are you up against?
  What obstacles are in the way? What blocks your path?
  It is important to speak about blocks in the language of "challenges" instead of "problems."

- **Strategies to Meet the Challenges:** Ways to overcome the hurdles that are blocking you presently.
Co-Create strategies to adjust and to bend without breaking from the commitments made in the plan. For example: when under a work deadline I will make my exercise session briefer, but not skip it.

Wellness Map Tool

Date: _____

All aspects of our lives are connected and affect one another. As we work on our relationships the workplace feels the positive outcomes. As we build strength at the gym we also build confidence and inner fortitude to complete a job. Use the Wellness Map Form to chart your own success. It is the agreement with yourself that brings clarity to what you desire to accomplish and creates a reference for you and your coach. Use your Well Life Vision and Areas of Focus to guide the way.

WELLNESS MAPPING 360™
METHODOLOGY

Name: _____   **Coach:** _____

Focus Area/ Change desired	Readiness? (1-5 scale with 5 being the most ready)	Action Steps	Indicators of Success	Who will Support You?	Accountability	Completion
(Attain a healthy weight)		1.	1.			
		2.	2.			
		3.	3.			
		1.	1.			
		2.	2.			
		3.	3.			
		1.	1.			
		2.	2.			
		3.	3.			

Comments:

Focus Area: What you want to change or accomplish?
How ready are you? How ready are you to make the changes you have identified? Rate your readiness on a 1-5 scale with 5 being the most ready.
Action Steps: The steps that will walk you to your desired change.
Indicators of Success: These are the mile markers along your path to reaching your desired changes and Well Life Vision

Wellness Mapping 360 ® Tools for Living Well   *Copyright 2004 Real Balance Global Wellness Services llc*

FIGURE 8.4

Sources of Support—Who can go on this journey with you, to help you out? State specifically who/what are your sources of support, encouragement, and accountability as you follow your wellness map into new territory? Encourage your client to think outside their typical or normal set of family and friends.

Realistic Goal Setting

Clients sometimes are very good at goal setting. Other times they may set their sights either too high or too low. For a wellness plan to have a chance, the goals have to be:

- Realistic and obtainable. (Can your client make these behavioral changes in a realistic and timely manner?)

- Short enough in terms of completion time for success to have a sufficiently timely reinforcing effect. (Quicker success = greater reinforcement. Take baby steps)

- Imperative enough that the person really wants to succeed in this area.

- Imaginable. Your client has to be ready and able to see themselves succeeding in that area.

- Specific. Keep it simple, to the point, and, as the British say, "Spot on!"

- Client generated. The goal has to be the client's goal for themselves, not the coach's goal for the client.

- Challenging. Difficult enough to bring out the best in your client but not so challenging that it works against your client.

> *I have never been lost, but I will admit to being confused for several weeks.*
> —Daniel Boone

Readiness for Change – Prochaska's Model

Part of selecting the Areas of Focus for the Wellness Map is best done through putting readiness for change theory into practice. The coach unfamiliar with this concept would profit greatly from studying it.

A foundational concept that is used pervasively in the wellness field, is the readiness for change work of James Prochaska and his associates, John Norcross, and Carlo Diclemente (*Changing For Good*). Used by thousands of addiction treatment programs and wellness programs world wide, Prochaska's work has had a profound impact. Deceptively simple at first, Prochaska reminds us that people don't change until they are ready to. While this seems absurdly obvious, when you examine most healthcare or treatment programs, you see that the healthcare provider often demands change immediately. The coach can also make this mistake.

Change is not controlled by a toggle switch that flicks on or off just because we—the healthcare provider, or the coach—see the need for change. Even if the client intellectually sees the need for change too, will it automatically happen? In fact, a real caution for coaches is not to rush to action. Many coaches are trained to respond quickly to their client's insightful statement with "So! What are you going to do about it?" When we rush to action in the arena of the lifestyle change process we are often sabotaging success and the client's ability to gain true insight.

When we plug the readiness for change theory into our coaching we can see that a client moves through the six stages that Prochaska outlines.

1. **Pre-contemplation.** The client is unaware and isn't concerned.

2. **Contemplation.** Client becomes aware and begins to consider change.

3. **Preparation.** Client begins exploring change possibilities (looks for resources, accessibility, affordability, etc.).

4. **Action.** Client takes action for change.

5. **Maintenance.** Client works at maintaining the change.

6. **Termination.** The new behavior is now a part of their life.

The wellness coaching client can be at a different stage of readiness in each specific behavior we look at. Just because someone is ready to exercise doesn't mean they are ready to quit smoking. We move and grow sequentially but not necessarily evenly.

All too often we approach results in lifestyle change in an all-or-

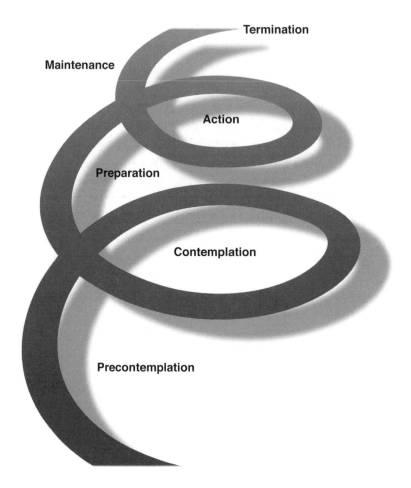

STAGES OF CHANGE

FIGURE 8.5

nothing manner. It is easy to conclude that our coaching failed if we don't see the person quickly succeed in accomplishing their lifestyle change and health goals. When we plug in the stages of change approach we may see that many times we are doing our coaching job very well when we help a person to simply advance along this change process. The client who is oblivious about their sedentary lifestyle, becomes aware of it, and merely begins to search out information about movement is, in fact, being quite successful at making progress in lifestyle change. Sometimes masterful coaching has taken place when we help a client move up one or two stages in this change process. Results need to be measured in the light of movement toward the goal or life-style change. The client and those administering a wellness coaching program need to be aware of the cycle of change and its specific use in lifestyle change.

Prochaska has found that this six-stage model is, in fact, a spiral model. People cycle and recycle through it. Perhaps someone contemplates beginning a program of recreating more with their children and prepares for it by buying some sporting equipment. Then their child cancels out of the outing by opting to go to an event with their own friends. The parent is disheartened and gives up trying to connect with their child, slipping back into contemplation, or even pre-contemplation. Perhaps they see their coach, realize it doesn't serve them to take the "rejection" so personally, and follows through with a wonderful time spent enjoying that planned for activity with their child at a later date.

Prochaska's Stages of Change and Coaching

The work of Prochaska and his associates is a deep and powerful resource. His trans-theoretical model of change matches therapeutic interventions with the appropriate stage of readiness for change. Here is an overview of ways to adapt the Stages of Change Theory to coaching.

1. Pre-contemplation. The person has no thought of changing, now or later. Others who care about them may repeatedly urge them to take action to improve their lives, but at this stage, they are truly deaf to their pleas. This is not resistance, just complete lack of awareness. A medical example would be someone who has high blood pressure but doesn't know it. Perhaps at a blood pressure screening at a health fair they discover their high numbers and move into Contemplation.

> **COACHING NOTE**
> The initial exploration and assessment phase of coaching can often help a person to shake out of this lack of awareness about a particular behavior or behaviors. Use of informal and formal wellness assessments often jog the person into awareness.

2. Contemplation. The person is thinking about changing—considering it, but can be quite ambivalent. "When in doubt, don't act." Introspection about why one follows a bad habit, what its payoff is, bringing both the rational mind and the emotions into play, helps to move the client to the next step.

> **COACHING NOTE**
>
> The contemplator can often stay here forever weighing the pros and cons. The coach approach helps the person examine how their current behavior is working for them, or against them. It offers them an ally—the coach—to help them move forward. The ultimately critical area of motivation, both internal and external is explored.

3. Preparation. Getting ready to change. Gathering information about topics and/or resources (Is there a pool/yoga class/hiking trail/bike path nearby?) Some preparatory steps might include: removing temptations, planning how action will be taken and arranging support and understanding from family, friends, perhaps a support group. When arranging substitutes for the missed habit or activity or substance, beware of substituting a new problem (over-eating, over-spending) for the old.

> **COACHING NOTE**
>
> Helping a client move from contemplation to preparation can be a huge accomplishment. Many times we feel we fail when we can't get a contemplator to jump into action. The new action can be the preparatory steps of gaining information, etc. Agreements to do so can be developed in the coaching process and methods of accountability set up so follow through is maximized by the client.

4. Action. The stage most of us picture, actual practice of the new way of being.

> **COACHING NOTE**
>
> The coach is in the ideal position to insure that the action taken is one that the client feels is entirely congruent with who they are, and how ready for change they are. Coaches can challenge the forever-preparing client to take action at a level they believe will work and then be a strong support during the process. Coaching accountability methods insure greater follow through. When the client fails to follow through, exploration of motivation can be of vital importance.

5. Maintenance. The actual process of maintaining the action that has been taken. Remembering that the Stages of Change Model is a *spiral* model—people frequently attempt a change, and then spiral back into earlier stages. Prochaska shows that many people benefit from learning the difference between a lapse and a total relapse, (a complete collapse back into the old way). Being prepared to recognize a lapse and take immediate action can save the effort and self-criticism.

> **COACHING NOTE**
>
> The wellness coach can play a vital role of support and accountability here. Often the client has never been successful at maintaining a change by themselves. Having a true ally in their coach, their chances of success improve dramatically. When the client spirals back to an earlier stage of a particular behavior, the coach can follow this process and help the client to re-set their goals based on the stage they are now in. A critical step in successful maintenance is self-monitoring or tracking our behavior. Through coaching the client sets up ways to keep track of how consistent they are being in their new behavior and avoids self-deception.

Recycling—back to one of the previous stages. *Changing for Good* shows that it is entirely possible for a person to fail at one stage or another, only to make a second or subsequent attempts that succeed.

6. Termination. The behavior has become a regular part of the person's life. Without much effort or thought, they naturally, and regularly engage in the new behavior. Depending on the desired change and the person, total termination of the problem behavior may not occur. Instead, there may be a lifetime of careful maintenance. In other cases, the problem is conquered and temptation to renew the poor behavior ceases. The Prochaska, et.al., state that the confidence that one has really succeeded peaks after a year but that temptation continues for two or three years.

> **COACHING NOTE**
>
> The coaching process helps the person to know when they have achieved their goal. The coach helps the client make distinctions between termination and on-going maintenance. The coaching process helps the client focus on other behaviors they are working on and/or helps them become clear about what they want to work on next. Coaching helps the client work towards independence and self-sufficiency and the termination of coaching as well.

How the Coach-Approach Honors Level of Readiness for Change

When you combine the wellness coach mindset with the readiness for change concept, you find that the coaching principles of asking permission, the wisdom of the client, and co-creation serve the client beautifully in the coaching process. In order to truly match the readiness-for-change stage where the client is with the coaching you do, you continually ask permission to explore into new areas. You respect the wisdom of the client, knowing that the answers lie within them, and they know what they are ready for much better than you do. Together you co-create a way to mutually explore a behavior and which one of the six stages of readiness for change they are in.

Three Steps for Coaching for Readiness For Change

1. Help your client recognize the stage of readiness they are in for specific behaviors.
2. Coach for completion of the client's current stage.
3. Coach the client toward the next step in the spiral model of change.

   Desire is the starting point of all achievement, not a hope, not a wish, but a keen pulsating desire which transcends everything.

   —Napoleon Hill

Achieving Buy-In and Commitment with Your Client

I've often told people that I like to work with clients who are ready, willing and able. Now for the willing part, what makes a person ready? Fully equipped, map in hand, guide at your side, what is it that allows clients, perhaps even urges them, to take that first step on the mountain's path? Contrary to some people's approach, giving your client a shove in the back is probably not a good idea. That first step has to come from within.

So what sells a client on lifestyle change? How and why do they buy-in to this notion? How does the notion become a commitment? How does lifestyle improvement become a genuine desire on the part of the client?

Perhaps some of the answers lie in whether your clients value themselves. As we stated briefly in Chapter Three (The Ten Tenets of Wellness), self-esteem is a critical factor in wellness. A person will do little for self if they do not care very much about themselves. If your client's feelings of self-worth are extremely low, they may benefit from counseling or therapy. For most everyone though, accessing that desire to live a better, more rewarding life comes from that reservoir of good feelings they have about themselves.

You will most likely not be able to help your client work through all of their self-worth/self-esteem issues before you begin implementing a wellness program. We all have to start somewhere. Sometimes a person has to begin by "acting as if," and that can be perfectly OK.

The client needs to see the benefits of the self-improvement efforts. "What's in it for me?" is the main question. A health educator would list the many good reasons for lifestyle improvement for a client, while the coach asks the client to come up with the answers themselves, and explores it with the client. If your client sees no particular benefits, or isn't aware of any, you might seek an agreement with them to research the area, or you might prime the pump by suggesting some benefits that you are aware of from wellness and medical research.

James Prochaska promotes the idea that when people see the benefits of a behavior, the barriers to that behavior are lowered. He believes that one way we stay stuck in the contemplative stage of change is that we underestimate the value of a particular behavior (like exercise) and overestimate the cost (time, effort, expense, etc.) of the change. By challenging your client to really look at a contemplated behavior change, in realistic detail, you may have a very productive coaching session where your client begins to see that the change is worth it. You can also strategize with them to lower the costs by coming up with ways of completing their goals that are easier and still very effective.

When you are being an effective coach you walk a very delicate and thin line between facilitating change and growth, and convincing someone of the benefits of growth. Remember, you are not in sales. A pull to become the salesperson is probably a tip that you are not honoring the principles and the stage of readiness of your client. An athletic coach can challenge a young woman or man to bring out a better game from the abilities that the coach sees and believes they have. However, the coach cannot make the player love the game and want to be out there on the field or court, playing with heart.

Keep all of your wellness coaching in the context of personal growth and development. When your client begins to see that their lifestyle changes are not just burdensome tasks, but instead, are ways of actualizing their own potential, motivation shifts into a completely different, and higher, gear. As I've seen clients become turned on to their own personal growth journey their excitement fuels a true passion to learn, to experiment and, ultimately, to grow! They become hungry for more information about what they can do to live richer, fuller lives. Their level of self-efficacy reaches an all-time high.

Early on, the wellness field grew out of the human potential/self-actualization movement. As the field has evolved some of us have become caught up in the wonderful world of research and statistics, etc., and forgotten what we can use that good data for. Your clients benefit the most when your coaching mindset is grounded in the values of personal growth. Let yourself wonder, "What if Abe Maslow had known about coaching?"

Motivation: Fear Based and Development Based

My first job as a counselor, after I got my Master's degree, was to be a caseworker in a residential treatment facility for emotionally disturbed adolescents. I found out then and there something that would prove to be true everywhere in life. I can't make anybody do anything. All I can do is invite.

As a wellness coach, remember that you cannot motivate anyone. You can, however, help them to find the motivation that resides inside of them. You can invite. You can help create the container, the situation of support. You can provide the presence of the conditions needed to facilitate personal growth. You can celebrate and reinforce when motivation shows up.

While there can be some value to the fake it until you make it approach, I would rather listen to Wayne Dyer talk about "You'll see it when you believe it." That brilliant little twist and play on words really does drive home the message that our internal beliefs shape our reality.

So, how do we coach people to discover their own motivation to be well? Public health campaigns, health educators, teachers, preachers, and parents have all tried very hard to convince us all to be healthy. We've seen programs and campaigns based on scaring us to be well (e.g., pictures of diseased lungs). We've been lured with incentives, cajoled by peer norms, shamed, blamed, ridiculed, seduced, tempted and much more. Some of it has worked. Some of it got us started, but not nearly enough of it was effective enough to sustain our lifestyle changes for most of us. Most of industrialized western society is still faced with lifestyle choice-related health concerns that statistically, at least, seem out of control.

Looking at the field of wellness and health-promotion, the work of Abraham Maslow (*Self-Actualization Theory*), Jay Kimiecik (*The Intrinsic Exerciser*), Gerry Jampolsky (*Love Is The Answer*), cancer-survivor Greg Anderson, and others, we can gain much wisdom about human motivation and behavior change. With this perspective in mind, let's consider basically two types of motivation: fear based and development based.

> *Frankly, helping people find the joy or passion in movement is what's missing from most . . . programs . . . Intrinsic motivation— performing a task primarily for its own sake is the most powerful way to change behavior . . .*

> —**Jay Kimiecik,** *The Intrinsic Exerciser*

What Motivates Us?

There are two types of fear-based motivation. Deficiency-based and threat-based. Deficiency-based motivation comes from a perception of lack, or what is missing in life. With the modern emphasis on youth, we see millions of people striving for ways to reclaim their youthful appearances. There is a widespread fear of the natural aging process. The anti-aging marketplace is enormous. Can a fear of growing old, or at least looking old, motivate a wellness lifestyle successfully?

Is wellness simply the postponement of morbidity? According to this point of view we're all mortal and will die someday, and since the human body does break down over time, being healthy as much as we can, for as long as we can, is all we can do!

Deficiency-based motivation shows up in shoulds. "I should exercise today because if I don't I'll lose my figure." "I should eat this horrible tasting stuff because I've made an agreement with my coach to eat it five times a week!" Yes, even coaching can become part of this army of shoulds that a person experiences. This is what Jay Kimiecik calls identified regulation. The person is not doing something because they truly want to do it, but because they've set up an external source of pressure, which the coaching relationship could unfortunately be a part of.

When your client speaks in imperative terms—"I have to . . ." or "I should . . ."—you might challenge them to ask themselves, "Who says?" Where is the message coming from that they should look a certain way, act a certain way, etc.? This might help them discover and discuss with you the pressures they feel from their family, their workplace, their subculture, their ethnic culture, etc. to be a certain way. Help them examine this and decide how they want to respond to this pressure from outside sources. Help them move from the imperative to the volitional. A large part of coaching is reminding people that they have choices.

Threat-based motivations can propel us to take action. These fall into the categories of known threats, unknown threats, illness avoidance and environmental threats. When we look for motivation for lifestyle changes, doing something to avoid pain, disability or illness would seem obvious enough. People who smoke know that the risks of cancer and heart disease are high. People who eat at fast-food restaurants several times every week and pile on the fatty-greasy-salty-sweet diet usually know that it is not good for them. These are known threats, backed up by tons of research. Threats can be where the people involved often know other people who have died of lung cancer or other diseases directly related to their behavior. Clearly, just knowing about the threat is often not enough.

One of the weaknesses of fear-based motivation is that human beings are remarkable at exercising ways to dodge it. Most of it is called denial and minimization. I like to say that many of us, when we do this dance of denial, like to use a little voodoo to insure our safety. We say magic phrases like "It will never happen to me." Or, "It will be all right." We are playing the probabilities here aren't we? Everyone seems to know or have known some person who lived a reckless life of smoking, drinking, overeating or being a couch potato, and lived to a ripe old age and enjoyed much of it. When we say "Oh, one more won't hurt me." how well are we really keeping track?

Old school health education programs tried the fear-based approach. We found that frightening people away from risky behavior does not work well over all. While fear-based motivation may get you started, it does not do well at sustaining change over time. We often witness this when someone has a teachable moment in the doctor's office. They receive a diagnosis and a dire warning. They listen. It gets their attention and the person takes some action to change their health behavior. The bigger challenge is continuing to behave in the healthier new way.

Sometimes your client may be motivated by the fear of developing a life-threatening illness. "I don't want to die young of heart disease like my Dad did." "I don't want to come down with diabetes like my Mom did." That fear may motivate them to lace up their walking shoes, or jump into the swimming pool more often. If it is working for your client, there may be no need to challenge it. Will it be enough over the long haul?

In wellness coaching we are usually not working with the people who succeed on their own at lifestyle change. We are more often working with people who have tried and failed, tried and failed a number of times by themselves. They need something new and different. Instead of someone reminding them to take their medicine, do their sit-ups, and eat their oat bran so they won't die sooner, how about an ally who helps them discover how living well is about joy, more energy, and more fulfillment?

Development-Based Motivation

Development-based motivation is really personal-growth motivation. Here we look beyond the deficiency needs that Maslow described in his theories—motivation and self-actualization. Now we look at what he called being needs. This is a view of human behavior that rests on the theory that all of us have within us a need to actualize our potential. When you see your clients removing the blocks that hold them back in their lives, they bloom. They flower into the amazing human beings they really are. Life coaches have long recognized this as the ultimate outcome of successful coaching. As a wellness coach, you support your clients in the same expression of self-actualization, on a whole-person, mind-body-spirit scale.

While all of this sounds rather idealistic and grand, it is also very concrete and practical in approach. The external sources of this motivation come, to a large extent, from the peer health norms that surround our client. As we described this concept briefly in The Ten Tenets of Wellness (Chapter 3), positive peer health norms can reinforce healthy behavior and can, in fact, open the doors for us to behave that way to begin with.

Coaching our clients to build strong and positive support systems made up of people who reinforce a healthy lifestyle can be some of our most valuable work. Every week our client's peers are around them much more than we are! It is so much easier to be active physically when our friends like to live that way too. Our clients can adopt new healthy behaviors more easily when they are surrounded by at least a few peers who already behave that way. Helping our clients expand connectedness in their lives may insure the adoption of, and the continuation of, healthy behaviors.

Another external, positive motivator can be the environment the person lives and works in. Living in a crowded, polluted, unsafe neighborhood can be a real threat to one's health, and make it difficult to engage in healthy new behaviors. On the other hand, a friendly, safe, clean neighborhood where there is access to healthy resources can make the adoption of new healthy lifestyle behaviors much easier.

Jay Kimiecik, in his book *The Intrinsic Exerciser*, contends that some of our best motivation comes from the inside-out. It is an outer expression of an inner motivation…that internal drive to be more of

Motivation—Intrinsic & Extrinsic

FEAR-BASED

Type 1: Deficiency-based

Comes from a perception of lack; operates on a sense of what is missing in life.

Internal Sourced

Need fulfillment—deficiency needs (Maslow)

Trying not to die—overcome the deficiency of lost health

Shoulds—internal pressure we put on ourselves

Identified regulation—sheer self-discipline we impose

External Sourced (Extrinsic)

Socio-cultural learnings

Norms, myths we are affected by

Identified regulation—doing it because you are supposed to, possibly even under agreement with a trainer/coach

Type 2: Threat-Based

Known threats

Unknown threats

Illness Avoidance

Environmental threats

DEVELOPMENT-BASED

Personal Growth-Based

Need fulfillment—being needs (Maslow)

Self-actualization

Human Potential

Internal drive to be more

Integration—seeking wholeness/completion

Love-Based

Movement to express love

Movement to protect that which is loved

Movement to receive love

Extrinsic or External Sourced

Positive peer health norms

Positive environmental conditions (safe, clean, friendly neighborhood, smoke-free public and workplaces)

Intrinsic or Internal Sourced

Inside-Out (Kimiecik) Motivation is from the inside first.

Joy/Pleasure

Satisfaction

Desire

Stimulation—It just feels good!

FIGURE 8.6

who we truly are . . . that seeking of expression of our wholeness and completeness. It is the intrinsic reward that is right there in the experience of the activity itself.

Why do you dance? Well, one person's answer might be: "I dance when I have to, like at a relative's wedding." Why do you play golf? Someone might answer: "I play golf because it's how I can build business relationships." Contrast that with the people who answer: "I dance because I love the feeling of movement! I love to move to the music! It's fun!" "I play golf because there is sheer joy when I hit a shot just right down that beautiful green fairway. I get so much satisfaction and relaxation out of it."

The first two people are operating on the external shoulds and real extrinsic deficiency motivation. The second pair are dancing and playing golf because they love it! Their motivation is intrinsic.

People with no experience of wilderness canoeing are sometimes baffled as to why my son, his best friends, and I, love to go deep into the northcountry on canoeing and fishing trips. When they hear our stories they pick up on the hardships of long days paddling, heavy packs and canoes on portages, mosquitoes, sleeping on the ground, etc. The pictures we bring back of big fish we've caught don't appear to be worth the sacrifice. What they can't know until they have experienced it are the more intrinsic rewards: the feel of the canoe slicing through still water, driven by only our own muscle power; the deep tranquility that can be found on the motorless lakes that we travel into; the amazing sense of brotherhood (or sisterhood) and self-sufficiency that we attain when we rely on each other and carry everything we need together.

So many unhealthy behaviors have immediate reinforcement! Nicotine imparts its effect on the smoker almost at once. Sugar tastes great as soon as the taste buds can perform their task. The tug of the couch into lethargy is pulling us down . . . now! The benefits of many healthy behaviors (e.g. exercise, good diet, etc.) are experienced further down the road. Our challenge in wellness coaching is to help our clients to have faith that the effort will be worth it. We reinforce immediately the desired behaviors, or help them set up ways of reinforcing it in the present. We also strongly support them in their vision of a healthy and vibrant life for them and help them hold that vision in their hearts and minds.

In effective wellness coaching, motivation is not about intellectually convincing someone of the benefits of a particular behavior, and then expecting them to agree and do! Wellness lifestyles may have an intellectual component, but wellness lifestyles are not often built simply on intellectual decisions. Clients benefit from looking deeper into their own motivation and trying methods that facilitate their own desire.

Kimiecik shares some research from a Canadian study, done by the Canadian Fitness and Lifestyle Research Institute, that found people who exercise regularly look to four primary sources of motivation:

- Fun, enjoyment, stimulation

- A feeling of accomplishment

- The pleasure of learning

- A concrete benefit, such as sleeping better and feeling calmer.

Help your client to explore a new behavior from the inside out. What is their experience in doing the behavior? What do they imagine it will be like to do that behavior when their body is more used to it, or they are more familiar with it? Help them discover the intrinsic joys in movement, in the sense of taste (help them find healthy foods they actually love the taste of), in their feeling of accomplishment. Help them find healthy lifestyle behaviors that pay off now in benefits they can feel, see, taste, hear, smell and touch.

Love or Fear

An ancient piece of wisdom that is often quoted by Gerry Jampolsky (*Love Is The Answer*) is that "everything we do comes either from love or from fear." A moment of reflection shows us what a truism this is. Think about an experience you may have had where a person was snobbish towards you. What were they afraid of? They certainly didn't appear afraid. Well, a snob is trying to be very selective about who and what they experience in their world. They are trying to make their world very small. How safe do they really feel? Their snobbish behavior said more about them than it did about you.

We've looked at lifestyle motivation that is based in fear. What about lifestyle motivation that is based in love? Some of our attempts to improve our lifestyles may come from our love for others. The grandparent who swims four times a week because they want to be around for their grandchildren (and take them swimming!). The couple who stopped smoking because their pet dog developed a lung problem from their second-hand smoke!

Coach your clients to explore who else would benefit from their improved lifestyle. Have them list their loved ones, friends and associates, and write down how these people would gain from them being healthier, more accessible, more active and vibrant! The airline steward/stewardess speech "put the oxygen mask on yourself first, and then assist others" is always a good reminder of one of the very best reasons to take care of yourself first; so you can be there, healthy and well, for others as well as for yourself.

Jay Kimiecik points out how as we develop mastery in a new exercise-related skill, we achieve a sense of accomplishment. That feeling of mastery bolsters our self-confidence and self-esteem. It feels wonderful to hit the ball down the middle of the fairway. It feels great to flow from one dance move gracefully into another. It feels great to run your first non-stop mile! This sense of accomplishment can be viewed as another form of self-love.

Self-love is once again what we are back to. Our client may start out at a place where they are willing to work their wellness plan for the sake of others, while they would not do it just for themselves. Hey! It's a start. As their health improves their feelings about themselves are likely to improve as well.

The Non-negotiable Law of Developmental Motivation

Greg Andersen, a cancer-survivor and author, reminds us of a truth that helps us understand this quest for self-improvement and self-actualization better. Instead of constantly striving and never arriving consider the following.

The essence of the law is this: I am complete but not finished. This is a statement of powerful truth. You are complete, whole, and fully alive right now! You need no more for life to be happy. You can be completely fulfilled with what is, now.

We are complete now, yet our natural development calls for further growth. This shift in thinking is critical. Lack becomes impossible. When we can see the inevitability of growth and change, we begin to become motivated by our dreams, not our deficiencies.

> *Satisfied needs, be they physical, psychological, or spiritual,*
> *do not motivate. Only unsatisfied hungers move people.*
> *This is one of the most powerful understandings we can have*
> *of ourselves and of others.*

> —Greg Anderson

Wellness coaching works best when we truly become allies with our clients and help them find motivation in development-based approaches. Exploring and listing all the ways in which the desired lifestyle changes fit into this approach provides motivation for change.

Motivation That Pulls You Forward
The Well-Life Vision

We've honored that fact that fear can get us started, but all too often does not sustain it's motivational qualities. Running away from the "Grim Reaper" seems a fear that diminishes as we continue to get by in life. What if, instead of looking over our shoulder in fear, we looked ahead and felt drawn towards what we truly want? The question becomes "What are you running toward that pulls your forward?" So if powerful motivation comes from a more positive psychology approach, more in line with what is truly desirable for our client, how can we help them to crystalize this?

Lasting lifestyle change is not about setting a goal and achieving it. It's about living our lives in the most health-enhancing way possible for the rest of our lives. So when we look ahead it's not just looking over the first hill to the next 10K race we run, or the day we quit smoking, it's looking over that ridge at a landscape that goes on forever (in mortal terms anyway!). So instead of a goal, even if it's a healthy one, we're talking about a vision of living the way we really want to live, living our best life possible. We want to stand on the ridge, so to speak, and look ahead saying "Yes! That's where I want to go!" And...we move into that landscape with our first step. For a Well-Life Vision to truly motivate it needs to be something we feel we can attain and start creating now, not when we retire and move to Shangra-La someday.

Holding that vision in our minds we can see that in order to attain it, we need to begin living our best life possible right now. We identify what those first steps on this journey are and begin our lifestyle changes now.

Coaching for Greater Self-care/Self-permission

As a wellness coach you may at times become very puzzled at the difficulty your client finds in behaving in new ways that are healthy for them. While they are completely equipped with knowledge, insight, awareness, accessibility, affordability, environmental support, and even a really good coach like you, they still won't give themselves permission to engage in the new behavior! In attempting to answer our golden question of coaching and wellness, "Why don't people do what they know they need to do for themselves?" self-permission is a indispensable concept.

Sitting in the shoes of that very puzzled coach I have asked my clients, "How did you hold yourself back from doing what you said you wanted to do this week?" They often say something like the following: "I don't know. I just forgot about it completely once we talked about it." "I had the time written down, just like we talked about, to go and workout, and then I thought I'd better get more housework done first." "Whenever I take the time to workout it feels like I'm taking time away from somebody else, like my kids, my partner, my job." "I feel really guilty when I just sit there and relax, — like I'm not getting anything done!" "My family always taught us to get all of our work done first before we could have fun, but now, as an adult, the work is endless!" "Are you kidding? Men (women) in my culture just don't do stuff like that!"

On one level or another, the client is denying himself or herself permission to exercise, relax, have fun, and express themselves, etc. They honestly don't feel all right doing these wonderful self-care, lifestyle-enhancing behaviors that they have intellectually concluded are good and important for them to do for their health. They are buying into a belief system, which may deny them needed gratification in any of a number of important areas of their lives. They may deny themselves adequate sleep, exercise, nutrition, contact with others, creative self-expression, and just plain enjoyment of life.

At times we need to help a client go back into the area of self-exploration and develop some understanding of where these powerful injunctions (as the Transactional Analysis theorists call them) come from. The roots for this may go deep. They tend to stretch back to four primary areas:

1. Self-esteem

2. Values, beliefs, and cultural norms

3. History of the person and their family

4. Myths and magical/irrational thinking

Self-permission and self-esteem beg the question, "Am I worth it?" The client debates with themselves "Am I worth the time? Shouldn't I be doing something for someone else (who is more worthy than I) instead?" As stated before, if the client's self-worth is extremely low, if self-hatred is more the issue, then, by all means refer this client to the help they need in a counselor's office.

For many clients gaining some insight about how they have ad-opted, without much examination and conscious choice, a set of val-ues and beliefs that were expressed in the norms of their family, their culture, and subculture can be very freeing. And yet we are not talking about a deep analysis of every bio-socio-cultural contributor to one's life. Instead, help your client to realize and acknowledge some of the historical factors that have made them who they are today, and then help them experiment with being different today. If repeated experi-ments (such as those you will see demonstrated in the case below) go nowhere in increasing self-permission it may be a hint to the client that there are old wounds that need counseling and therapy. It may be more about healing than coaching.

All-Work and No-Play

I have had numerous clients teach me great lessons about self-permission and self-denial. One client was a woman who grew up in a hard-working family from the Great Plains. Her pioneer grandparents and great-grandparents had set the tone for self-denial and self-sacrifice as a survival strategy. Their religious practices had reinforced and glorified this. Admittedly this way of living may have been quite realistic in the years that helped them make it through the great drought of the dust bowl years, and the economics of the Great Depression. However, for her parents and for her, this severe way of living did not mesh with the abundant, yet fast-moving and high-stress world that they found themselves in.

This client was a self-employed businesswoman who found herself living a life of all-work and no-play. She was extremely stressed, significantly overweight, and, despite a hard-working life of service to others, was both personally miserable and struggling with the viability of her business.

As we coached together and our alliance grew into one of sincere trust, I challenged her to do more self-care. Her level of self-denial was so great that it had been literally more than fifteen years since she had taken a vacation of any kind, and she could not remember the last live concert she had been to, despite absolutely loving music. She did not exercise at all, but I knew that this was not the first place to start.

Her first suggested coaching homework was to research the schedule of a concert venue within an easy drive of her home (about fifty prairie miles). She came to our next session excited to report that the Beach Boys were actually doing a reunion tour and stopping there. I challenged her to take the extreme (to her) act of buying tickets for her and her husband and go to it! Rocking at that concert was like pushing a wedge in the slightly opened door of self-care for her. Little by little she began to do more for herself.

Eventually she found that her neighbor had a Golden Retriever that wasn't getting enough exercise. She asked the neighbor if she could take the dog out walking regularly. This helped her give herself permission to take so much time for something so "unproductive" as walking. The neighbor was thrilled. She and the Retriever became good buddies and daily walks of at least an hour ensued. This

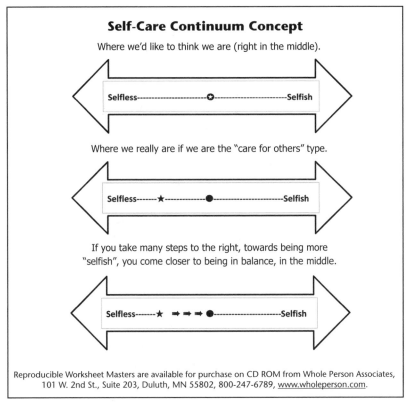

FIGURE 8.7

combined with a self-initiated participation in a dietary-support group helped the weight fall off of her, and the dog slimmed down, too!

Doing things for self, especially just for recreation and mere enjoyment felt really foreign to her at first. This was very incongruent with her view of herself and the world. To do even a little for herself she had to think in extremes and doing so helped her to grow!

Myths and Magical/Irrational Thinking

Some of what we learn in our families and in our communities and cultures as we grow up are really myths, yet we take them on as truth. Some are self-limiting beliefs that the group (family, peers, community) somehow taught as truisms. These falsehoods become seen as "just the way life is." This is the view of the world where there is a sense that we are powerless to prevent the inevitable, be it poverty, illness, misfortune or unhappiness.

In the economically depressed area where I grew up there was an unspoken message that a young person should not think that they are anyone special. It was OK to be OK, but not OK to be great! To strive for excellence was seen as an attempt to raise yourself above your peers and that was considered narcissistic. At least, that is how I came to interpret my experience and observations there. I saw my best friend, who I always thought was just as intelligent as me, if not more so in some areas, succumb to the message from his family not to see education as a vehicle to greater success or happiness. He was directly told to not even consider college. A job, the military…these were his only options. While no one but him can judge his own happiness and how it all worked out, I still wonder, "What if?"

Health myths in some families abound. "None of the men in our family live long." "All of the women in our family are overweight, it's just the way we are." This type of insidious programming takes place with a very low level of awareness of the consequences. In an attempt to protect us from the bitter disappointments of life, our families set us up to expect certain health outcomes as inevitable. This gives the whole family permission to behave in ways that probably usher in exactly what we fear. Why bother to exercise and eat right when we're going to die before fifty anyway?

The work of philosopher Sam Keen (*Your Mythic Journey*) is a valuable resource for understanding what he calls our own personal mythology. Understanding the myths that we live and die by is one of his valuable contributions to wellness.

Coach for possibility thinking with your client. Help them become conscious and aware of myths like those we have described above. Encourage to have them to talk with a number of friends and relations who may have received the same messages and see how everyone dealt with them in their own way.

Think impossible and dreams get discarded, projects get abandoned, and hope for wellness is torpedoed. But let someone yell the words, "It's possible," and

*resources we hadn't been aware of come rushing in
to assist us in our quest.*

—**Greg Anderson**

Affirming and Acknowledging the Positive

Most of us tend to overlook what we are doing right. We take for granted all the good things that we did during the course of the day. We take for granted our strengths, talents, and abilities. So seldom do we take time to honor what we are blessed with, or to honor what we have accomplished.

As coaches, part of honoring our client is to jump on the opportunity to affirm the positive when we see it in evidence. Clients need to hear it. They need to hear what a good job they are doing, even if, to them, they are just doing their job.

Affirmations made by the client can be powerful statements that take them closer and closer to their goal. By affirming that they are whole and complete they realize how that is true. By repetitively affirming that they are lovable and attractive, they become so to the rest of the world.

In recent years the Positive Psychology Movement has emerged and been very validating for the field of coaching. From it's inception in the mid-1980s, coaching has been a strengths-based approach that has constantly affirmed and acknowledged the positive. The work of Martin Seligman (*Authentic Happiness*) and others has provided evidence that shows we've always been on the right track.

A basic life coaching exercise that works extremely well with our wellness coaching clients is to suggest to them that each day they notice three things that they have done that they want to acknowledge themselves for and write them down. The act of writing down cements the acknowledgements more firmly. What is being acknowledged can be actions they have taken: "I acknowledge myself for using my calorie-counting app on my phone at all three meals today!" Or, they can acknowledge themselves for some aspect of their character that "showed up" and helped them with their wellness efforts. "I really give myself credit for having the courage to ask my boss about realistic work expectations."

Wellness Coaching and the Inner Critic or Gremlin

One of the greatest ways that we dis-empower ourselves is through allowing the inner-critic to rule. Each of us has a part of our thought patterns that we refer to as the inner-critic or the gremlin. Operating out of fear, this part of us vehemently holds to the status quo and fights change—even change that is good for us.

Some people say the inner-critic is just trying to protect us. Its idea of protection is like this. Think of a high-school age boy who goes to a dance. His number one fear is being rejected. So the inner-critic/gremlin protects him by insuring he will not be rejected. He never asks anyone to dance. Mission accomplished. No rejection. No dancing either!

The inner-critic is our inner-voice that speaks to our self-doubt and fear. When we listen to it we hear voices from the past that we have taken in, that tell us we aren't good enough, beautiful enough, smart enough, etc. The inner-critic tells us we don't belong out there being successful. The inner-critic destroys our confidence and causes us to withdraw from opportunities, or at least to perform poorly. At worst the inner-critic triggers all our negative feelings about ourselves, even self-loathing.

The key in gremlin fighting is to catch yourself early and not give the gremlin your ear. As you listen to it, it grows. Soon all you can hear is your voice of self-doubt and negativity. The other thing to remember about your inner critic is that you cannot kill it! It is really a part of you and will always make its attempt to gain your attention.

I worked with a professional golfer and helped him improve his game by silencing his inner-critic. Whenever he made a bad shot on the course his gremlin would attack him savagely! He would get so angry with himself that his next shot was almost guaranteed to be just as bad or worse. After great work on his part through our coaching he thought he had finally vanquished his cognitive nemesis and was appalled when it raised it's ugly head again on the course. "Wait a minute!" I said to him. "Are you waiting for the day when the gremlin doesn't come on the course with you?" "Well, yeah…" he replied. I had to tell him that that day would not come. The gremlin will always show up. Your challenge is to immediately recognize it, and silence it. You can do that effectively, but yes, it will always try. Giving yourself a hard time for not keeping your inner critic/gremlin in line is what I call advanced gremlin activity.

Rick Carson, author of *Taming Your Gremlin*, says that we are best off when we realize that the gremlin does not have our best interest at heart. We have to recognize when we are listening to the self-doubter within, and quickly silence it. Here is one method for doing just that.

Five "R" Process for Gremlin Fighting

1. RECOGNIZE when what you are saying to yourself is gremlin-talk.

   a. Know ahead of time what some of your Gremlin's favorite lines are.

   b. Distinguish between gremlin talk and good problem-solving reflection.

   c. Identify if this is a particularly gremlin-vulnerable time for you. Use the H.A.L.T. Self-Quiz (below)

2. REFUTE the gremlin talk.

   a. "This is *not* true. What's true for me is . . ."

   b. Don't get into a debate with your gremlin.

3. REMOVE the gremlin from your experience.

   a. Use your own favorite gremlin-removing fantasy (gag 'em, bind 'em, throw 'em in the dungeon and lock them up again!)

   b. Don't let the gremlin travel with you. Throw them out of the car, out of your workplace, or wherever you are.

4. REGAIN your self-confidence. Remember how you have been successful in the past and affirm your abilities and talents.

5. RETURN to the present. Focus on the here and now.

You will notice that one of the "Rs" of gremlin fighting is *not* reassure. Some clients like to believe that the gremlin is really their own inner hurt child who is always fearful and needs kindness, gentleness and reassurance. There is an important distinction to draw here. Your gremlin or inner-critic is not your inner child, it is the accumulation of lies and distortions of reality that frighten and weaken your inner child. The inner-critic is just that—a critic! It constantly criticizes our actions, decisions and even our feelings and labels them not as just ineffective, but as wrong and stupid.

When we engage in conversation with our gremlin, even if we think we are making peace or reassuring it that all is and/or will be OK, we give it attention, and it grows. When we really realize that the inner-critic bases its FEAR campaign on False Evidence Appearing Real, we realize that we are engaging in debate, conversation and relationship with a pack of lies.

A valuable little tool that I believe was originated in work from the addictions field is the H.A.L.T. Self-Quiz.

Whenever you have identified your Gremlin, or Inner-Critic as being active, or you seem to be starting the process of reviewing your entire life in retrospect. Ask yourself, am I:

Hungry?

Angry?

Lonely?

Tired?

If so . . . HALT! Stop the self-review process until you are no longer hungry, angry, lonely, or tired. It's not a good time to look back on your whole life.

One of the best ways that a wellness coach can continue to be of value to a client is to help them spot the gremlin when it shows up. Gently challenge your client to examine something that they have just said. "Could what you are saying be gremlin-talk"? "Does that sound like your inner-critic?"

There is amazing power in simply noticing. Awareness opens eyes, doorways, and lives. It is the automatic pilot style living of habit that dulls our awareness and limits our lives. It is the subtle way we begin listening to the old tape recordings of our inner-critic that brings out our fears and causes us to grind growth and progress to a frightened halt.

When we notice, when we sharpen our awareness to catch the gremlin in action and then employ the Five "R"process above, we shut it down early, before it can gain strength. Have a zero tolerance of the gremlin's presence. No negotiations with a pack of lies that masquerades as self-talk in our own heads.

As your client progresses through the stages of change the gremlin will grudgingly take the journey with them, complaining and attempting to sabotage progress all the way. In fact some of the ways I've been most helpful to my clients is when I've helped them see how it is often their very success that triggers the self-doubt, self-worth questions of the inner-critic. The gremlin gets really scared when you are being successful at change!

Your client may struggle with this concept of the inner-critic or gremlin. Recommend that they read the extremely insightful and entertaining little book by Richard Carson, *Taming Your Gremlin*. Have some coaching conversations around what they've learned and how it applies to them.

I free myself not by trying to be free, but by simply noticing how I am imprisoning myself in the very moment I am imprisoning myself.

—**Rick Carson**, *Taming Your Gremlin*

Working With What Works

Coaching brings to the field of wellness many effective and practical methods to help our wellness coaching clients find success in behavioral change. Here are some very concrete ways to work with your clients to help them make lifestyle improvements that last.

Structures

Adopting new habits that are healthy requires continual reminders. Our wellness consciousness can be stimulated by a variety of physical things coaches call structures. Structures are any kind of visible device that reminds us (or our clients) of our wellness vision, goals, or tasks.

Some good insightful work by a client of mine once produced the awareness that she was taking life much too seriously and that the lack of joy in her life really was affecting her stress-level and consequently her health and well-being. She vowed to adopt an attitude of lightness and to seek to see the humor, irony, and the up side of her daily events.

She knew that the workplace was her biggest challenge for this. I explored with her the type of image that always brightened her thoughts and feelings and found she loved clowns. While some people actually are frightened of clowns, they always brought a smile to her face. I asked if she had any small clown statuettes. She did and I asked her to select one and bring it to her desk at work.

Whenever she noticed the clown figure on her desk she was to immediately take a deep breath, and if possible at that moment, lighten her thoughts. As simple as it was, it worked! To ensure that it would continue to be effective I encouraged her to move the location of the structure on and around her desk area, or to bring in another different figure of a clown. This would freshen up the structure and stimulate her memory of her commitment to shift her consciousness to a lighter and brighter view.

Structures can include: photos or magazine clippings of places and events that are in line with one's wellness vision (such as an older person who still climbs mountains or a dream vacation destination that you want to be in shape for); photos of loved ones you want to be healthy enough to enjoy being with; little pieces of nature (rocks, seashells, etc.) that remind you of the active things you like to do in the natural world (such as hiking or snorkeling); photos or magazine clippings that show someone doing the activity or displaying the emotions or behaviors you want to emulate; something that to you (or your client) represents an important metaphor that was arrived at in a great coaching session. Unrealistic or perfectionistic images (such as super-model photos) don't work well as structures. Get creative with your client and brainstorm what would work for them.

Journaling

We spoke of journaling in Chapter 7, referring to it as a tool for exploration. It, and coaching itself, can help your client explore in ways beyond their own thinking.

Our own personal reflection has value, but it is limited, both in viewpoint (which always includes blind spots), and in what it brings forth. Talking with you, the coach (as well as others), allows for the power of relationship and requires your client to put their thoughts into words in order to be understood. This vastly different cognitive process allows them to synthesize their thinking and often yields entirely new perspectives and insights.

Writing their thoughts out on paper (or typing them onto our computer), draws upon yet another process that takes their reflections deeper and often in new directions that mere sitting and thinking would not reach. Journaling is another tool of elicitation. Engaging in the journaling process helps your client understand that all of this wellness/lifestyle improvement work is really about personal growth. Journaling helps them stay on task—the task of actualizing their potential and expressing their true nature.

Help your clients feel more attracted to journaling by urging them to do it their own way. Some people feel very intimidated by journaling. They sometimes think they have to journal like Henry David Thoreau. Support them in giving themselves permission to journal any way they find effective. Draw outside the lines. Be sloppy, be neat, it's up to them. They can use a structured, published journal or just write consistently in an inexpensive spiral notebook.

Journals need not be a simple chronology of events. They may at times just be a stream of consciousness. At other times they may be a gratitude list, or a list of action steps that were taken. Support your client in making their journal work for them, not the other way around.

Urge your clients to give their journal top security. A really secure journal allows them to say what they really need to say and express themselves. On their computer a password-protected electronic journal works well for this. Keep paper journals reliably secure and confidential.

Make journaling part of the coaching process by securing a commitment as to how often they will journal each week. A commitment to journaling seven days a week is usually a setup for failure. Go for four or five—maybe even three entries to start with. Challenge the client who suggests only once or twice a week.

Urge your client to have only one rule about their journaling . . . that they write it by themselves, with no help from their gremlin! The inner-critic will attempt to seize this opportunity too. Beware and be forewarned! Urge your client to identify when their thoughts are slipping into gremlin talk" and do what it takes to silence it. Also, urge your client to observe and be patient as they go through the change process.

Coaching With Your Journey to a Healthier Life

A companion journal to this book is *Your Journey to a Healthier Life: Paths of Wellness Guided Journals: Volume One* (by the author). Formatted as a personal journal this spiral-bound book allows your client to work with you (or is more self-directed, on their own) through the Wellness Mapping 360°™ process. Your client can write their own journaling, respond to powerful questions, create their Well-Life Vision and their Wellness Plan, and keep track of their behavior using a large number of tracking forms in the back. (Available from this same publisher.)

Tracking

Many of the behaviors that our clients seek to change can be tracked very easily. Frequency, intensity, duration and the nature of exercise can be written down, preferably each day it happens. Your client can gain much by writing down everything that they eat in a week. Most fitness programs provide charts for writing down both what you plan to eat and then what you actually do eat everyday. This is a very helpful process to teach a client the reality of their eating patterns, and then to improve them. There are also a number of commercial sites on the web that feature online diet journaling. Some of these are quite sophisticated and may appeal to some clients.

Simpler is better for some clients. One of the most effective tracking devices ever invented is the wall calendar. By having a wall calendar displayed in a frequently visible place in the client's home or workplace, they can quickly see their identified wellness behavior (or lack thereof) by marking on it with a heavy pen or marker.

The task of tracking raises awareness. It brings new consciousness to the process of change and helps the person be more accountable to themselves. It helps the person to see their improvements in black and white and celebrate them. It reduces self-deception and increases self-efficacy. It also allows the coach and client to know when goals are being reached and when they remain elusive.

If your client is somewhat tech-savvy they may love working any of the online and phone-based apps available to track their wellness activities and coaching efforts. Phone apps make burdensome tasks like calorie counting easy. Apps allow clients to record what they

Weekly Wellness Tracker

Name _____

Focus Area – Desired Health Outcome _____

Date _____

Action Steps	Check-in Plan	Monday	Tuesday	Wednesday	Thursday	Friday	Saturday	Sunday
1.								
Duration								
Comments								
2.								
Duration								
Comments								
3.								
Duration								
Comments								
4.								
Duration								
Comments								

What relaxation method did you use? (*circle one*) Nature • Music • Deep Breathing • Meditation • Yoga/Tai Chi • Guided Imagery • Other

How did you sleep this week? (*circle one*) Good • OK • Not well • Comments _____

How did you take care of yourself this week? _____ What disappointed you this week? _____

On a scale of 1-10 (10 being the best) how well did you do this week? What encouraged you this week? _____

1 • 2 • 3 • 4 • 5 • 6 • 7 • 8 • 9 • 10

What do you want to remember to talk over with your coach? _____

Reproducible Worksheet Masters are available for purchase on CD from Whole Person Associates, 101 W. 2nd St., Suite 203, Duluth, MN 55802, 800-247-6789, www.wholeperson.com.

FIGURE 8.8

have eaten, scan bar codes on food products, compare restaurant menu items, track workouts, chart their walk, run, or bike ride on a map using their built-in GPS and much more. While health and fitness apps (most of them free) have been downloaded millions of times, it's suspect how many are in use today! The key is to make the use of the apps part of the coaching. With some simple accountability clients can use these tools more consistently and successfully. Successes can be celebrated and a realistic picture of progress, or the lack thereof can be addressed. The world of fitness apps is constantly changing. See the Bibliography and Resources section of this book for a popular list.

Wellness Mapping 360°
Accountability & Support

There is more to accountability and support than first meets the eye. Here is the real roll up the sleeves part of wellness coaching. All the best-laid wellness plans will not produce results effortlessly. Add value to the coaching experience of your client by working shoulder to shoulder with them on core issues such as motivation, self-permission, and self-defeating thinking. Be ready with tools and ideas for them to try out that help them to work through whatever is in the way of a successful wellness journey.

Obtaining Loophole-Free Accountability

Once goals are set, how does the client follow through on them? Coaching is distinguished by its emphasis on accountability and providing the methodologies that help a client to attain high levels of it. When a coach holds a client accountable, they are really helping the client to be accountable to themselves. The coach works for the client, not the opposite. In your role as wellness coach you are there to co-create with the client agreements of accountability that serve that client well. I've found it critical to a client's acceptance of the accountability concept that they understand that <u>they</u> are not accountable to <u>you</u>. They are accountable to *themselves*.

The part of your client that is afraid of change will search for loopholes—ways out—contained in your agreements for accountability. Your client's gremlin or inner critic will be on alarm status as you co-create your agreements because it knows that accountability is serious stuff! It gets results!

For loophole-free accountability follow these guidelines.

1. Start with good goals nd well-thought-out Action Steps (using the guidelines above).

2. Match the degree of accountability to the client, the situation, and what they are asking for. Simply reporting back verbally at the next session may be entirely adequate for a specific Action Step with one client. Another Action Step in another situation, or with a very different client may require very stringent accountability. Ascertain what degree of accountability a client usually wants and needs in your foundation session with them, then keep observing and experimenting and see what really works.

3. Keep closing the escape routes. When a client is vague about when or how they will report back to you, require them to clarify it and nail it down. Help your client explore their "Yes, but…" excuses and see how valid they really are.

4. If they are having trouble committing ask your client what you should do if you don't hear from them by when they agreed. "What if I don't get your e-mail by the end of the day on Monday. What should I do?" Keep What if-ing them until you get a clear agreement.

5. Offer to connect but keep the responsibility on the client. "OK, if I don't get a response to my reminder-e-mail that I've sent back to you, what should I do?"

At the beginning of coaching we have to teach our clients how accountability can work and what we are and are not willing to do to help. When a client identifies an Action Step they want to take I often will say "How can I help you with that? How can I help you really get it done?" Of course they don't know what the options can be until I let them know.

Keep the responsibility on your client to remember to get things done. Agree to respond to their e-mails notifying you that they accomplished an Action Step, but don't drive yourself mad reminding all of your clients to perform all of these behaviors. Model good boundary setting. For example you might want to refuse to respond to e-mail over the weekend.

Encourage your client to find other sources of accountability also. Some of the best accountability is a walking buddy waiting outside your door early in the morning waiting for you to join them. Four-legged fitness trainers (dogs!) are amazing at consistent accountability! Evidence even shows that dog owners who walk their dogs are more fit than non-dog owners.

When Your Client Does Not Complete Action Steps

No shame, no blame. Your client is not reporting in to their boss, drill Sargent, or third-grade teacher. They are accountable to themselves. Sometimes "life happens" and gets in the way realistically. I suppose a dog really could eat a Wellness Plan!

Again, we want to keep the responsibility on our client. Explore the client's report on what happened and, if it seems appropriate to ask, you might say "So, how did you allow that to get in the way of completing your Action Step?" Our clients expect to be held to their word. They really do want to succeed by completing these Action Steps that they, themselves, co-created with you. They don't want a free-pass. When we jump in and rescue our clients we actually collude with them in staying stuck. "Oh, I know it's hard to do this." "It's okay. That's alright." This is not what our clients benefit from, or actually want to hear.

With your client chose to Reset, Recommit, or Shift. Perhaps the Action Step had too high a criterion. Instead of walking five days a week, reset to three. Recommit to the five times a week if the client feels like they are sure it's realistic for the coming week. Shift to a whole new Action Step if needed.

The key is to be the Ally not the Adversary. Keeping coming from a place of "All I'm doing is help you do what you really want to do."

Wellness Mapping 360°™
Ongoing Evaluation & Measurement

We've come a long way with our client on their wellness journey. As their success in making lifestyle improvements has continued they have ventured into previously unknown lands. Evaluation provides feedback. It asks "Are we on the right path? How are we doing?" Good coaching is always examining the road traveled and the results. We ask and we measure. We constantly seek to find the value in what we have done.

Self-Report Data

Check in with your client on a regular basis to process the process. Examine the coaching relationship and the coaching process at regular intervals. You both may have wandered off the trail you thought you were on or coaching may have become less effective and less satisfying even though nothing has been said about it.

Refer back to the wellness plan originally developed. Are you both in alignment on this process and moving towards these goals? Explore how your client feels about it, no matter what the numbers say.

One-to-ten self-ratings are very helpful. Asking a client to rate their progress on a particular behavior from a low-effectiveness of one, to a high-effectiveness of ten. This can itself be a tool of elicitation and uncover important material to discuss.

Biometrics and Measurements

Here again, wellness coaching works with many outcomes that we can measure concretely. Our clients can record their number of hours of sleep. They can work with their physician and other health-care providers to attain physiological measures that let us know whether we're on the right path, or not.

The biometric feedback that clients receive will always have a psychological effect. What the effect is, from jubilation to depression depends on our client and their belief system. Be sure to explore the feeling-impact of test results, physiological measurements of any kind. Evaluation on these variables can produce results that are encouraging or discouraging. Exploration of their impact on your client's motivation will be key. Talk about it and explore it, but also observe how your client responds behaviorally to it over the following weeks.

Using Inventories Again

One of the easiest ways to assess progress is to have the client re-take the particular wellness instrument that they took at the beginning of coaching. The Wellness Inventory and TestWell, and even regular HRAs are very well-suited for this. They produce well-organized data that can be used to re-set the course of coaching. Re-taking the Wheel of Life can produce rich coaching conservations.

Figure-Ground

As we attain a sense of completion in one area of focus it seems to lose energy and fades from our attention. What once was paramount and so important now recedes into the background. What to work on next becomes the big coaching question. An informal review of the wellness plan will help, but it may be most helpful for the coach to be sensitive to the shifts in energy, interest and excitement that they see in their client as they review new areas on to work. Follow the energy. What seems most pressing now and what is there motivation to work on? Looking at what is now primary in the person's life may help reset the course of wellness coaching for the client.

> *Overt action without insight is likely to lead to temporary change.*
>
> —**James Prochaska,** *Changing For Good*

Wellness Mapping 360°™
Clear Measurable Outcomes

How can our clients know when they have arrived at their destination? How can they answer the classic question from the back seat of the automobile "Are we there yet?"? When we may have never been there before, how can we know what the X-marks-the-spot on our pirate's wellness treasure map looks like?

Hopefully, at the onset of our quest, the destination was adequately described. The more measurable goals, like percentage of body fat reduction, are easy to determine. The more elusive destinations that depend on subjective self-assessment, may be just as valid, but now both the client and the coach may discover they are a bit foggy or tougher to recognize. To bolster your client's confidence and help them recognize success, lobby for at least some clear measurable outcomes in the wellness plan to begin with.

Maintaining Success & Managing Stress

When do we know that a new behavior has been integrated as part of the client's lifestyle? How will they know? Many improvements in lifestyle behavior relapse under stress. A smoker has kicked the habit until a project deadline at work coincides with the filing date for their taxes and the birthday of their child. An unexpected surgery means starting an exercise program all over again. Life happens!

Prochaska addresses the maintenance stage of change very well in *Changing For Good*. He points out how stress triggers the re-emergence of old behaviors (usually exactly the ones we've been working on changing), and so argues that we should build into our wellness plan some aspects of stress management.

Coach your client to develop the skills they need to cope with the inevitable stress that will challenge their progress. Co-create a back-up plan of action to use during times of extra stress. Realize that this may occur after coaching has already concluded, so your client needs to be self-sufficient in stress management strategies and skills.

Outcomes for The Client, The Coach and "Third Parties"

As we've said, our clients want to see concrete results. The coach also needs feedback about how well they have been coaching. Obtaining client-satisfaction reports from our clients can be extremely rewarding. Looking at cumulative data from our client list can be valuable. Listening to recordings of our coaching sessions, or better still, getting some mentor coaching along with it can help us improve our coaching like nothing else.

Many wellness coaches work in settings where they are either employed by a wellness coaching company (insurance, EAP, disease management, etc.) or are contracting for a company to provide coaching to employees. Those who are paying for the coaching want to know that it is effective. While not privy to the confidential information about any individual client, they can make excellent use of aggregate data to measure coaching's effectiveness. Again, this is where there's nothing like the concreteness of biometric data to make wellness coaching shine. Coaching programs are often evaluating changes in a client population's blood pressure scores, A1C scores (diabetes indicator), cholesterol scores, weight loss, percentage body fat, BMI, and more. They look at the effect on absenteeism, presenteeism (the degree to which you are at "present" and functional at work – for example back pain or headache will reduce presenteeism), productivity and employee turnover. The ultimate bottom line will be seeing how wellness coaching might (hopefully) affect healthcare costs in a positive way.

The Power of Habit

Many times I've worked with clients who have made up their minds to change. They have determined that a change is needed and they have decided to change an old habit of their behavior that has been around for a long time (such as overeating, being sedentary or smoking). They appear motivated to change and vow to stop a certain behavior from occurring any more.

Before long they are disappointed that the behavior that they decided to end had resurfaced once again. Often the client would be disappointed not only that the behavior was back, but disappointed in their own lack of will power. They had thought, contrary to what we've seen Prochaska teach us, that change was an event (a decision) not a process. They made it about strength of character and gave their own inner critic plenty to berate them with.

Don't underestimate the power of habit! Once we have adopted a new behavior there are actually neural pathways set up in our nervous system related to this behavior. Today's neuroscience tells us that our habits are part psycho-physiological! Our bodies, as well as our minds, are in the habit of reacting a certain way, so no wonder changing a habit is not as simple as making a resolution.

Urge your client to consider these quick tips for changing habits.

1. Practice patience. Research tells us that it takes as many as 180 days to truly drop an old habit and adopt a new one. So stay with it.

2. No beating yourself up! Don't put yourself down because you find yourself engaged in the old habit.
Be compassionate with yourself instead.

3. Celebrate catching yourself! Take the repetitions in stride. Realize that despite the old habit showing up again, you are committed to changing the habit. Instead of putting yourself down ("There I go again!"), celebrate the fact that you managed to catch yourself and become aware of it. As you catch yourself earlier in the practice of the old habit, you'll have even more to celebrate!

4. Use structures, as discussed on page 155, to help remind you of the new habits you want to adopt. Structures are little physical reminders that help you remember your goals. They may be little signs you print up for yourself reminding yourself to: "Wait to answer the call after 2 rings, not sooner!"; "Breathe!"; "Call a friend today!"; "30 min. of writing every day." Another hint about structures—move them around, change the look of them so they don't start blending in with the background again (out of habit!).

5. Involve others in your goals. Let co-workers, friends and family know what you are working on changing. Enlist their support and possibly their awareness and feedback to help you stay engaged in the habit changing process.

6. Get a coach! Working with a coach gives you someone to help you get clear about what behaviors you really want to change; give you support in the process and/or hold you accountable to do what you say you will do to change the habits.

Every man is more than just himself; he also represents the unique, the very special and always significant and remarkable point at which the world's phenomena intersect, only once in this way and never again.

—Hermann Hesse

Every person's path to and through change will be unique. As we strive to develop ways to help people make the lifestyle changes that will maximize their wellness we must remember that they are all just offerings we make for each person to examine for themselves.

Chapter 9

Choosing, Living, Loving, Being: Coaching the Strategic, Lifestyle, Interpersonal, and Intrapersonal Aspects of Effective Change

*Whatever course you decide upon, there is always someone
to tell you you are wrong. There are always difficulties
arising which tempt you to believe that your critics are
right. To map out a course of action and follow it to the end,
requires some of the same courage which a soldier needs.*

—Ralph Waldo Emerson

It's a big world out there. Before your coaching client lies so many possibilities! There are so many aspects to the journey that it may be overwhelming at times. There is a path to be found and chosen, there are things to explore and goals to set. So many choices to make that at some point an organizing process may assist us to proceed.

Imagine your client is struggling to find direction, feels unclear about what to do next, and is wandering in circles from one topic to the next. They are committed enough to the journey of change so they are working with you, yet they don't know where to start. Perhaps they are afraid to even take that first step. To return to our coach-as-mountain-guide analogy, do you simply follow your client patiently around through the trackless thick trees at the base of a mountain range? How can you best serve them as a coach, as a guide?

Throughout this book we've continually talked about the benefits of a holistic approach to growth and development. Yet, does holistic mean an inclusion of everything? You need an organizing methodology. As a coach, one way you can best serve your client is to have enough knowledge of change theory and development to offer a variety of ways that your client can look at the change process, embrace it and begin their journey with you by their side. You do this by keeping this knowledge in the back of your mind to guide you as you guide them. As a coach it helps you think on your feet and gives you a sense of what needs to be included in the work you are doing with the client.

One great contribution that coaching has made to the growth and development process or movement is that it is so focused and practical. It is not about the geological history of the mountains in front of you, it is about choosing a peak to climb, getting in shape for the challenge, loading your pack and having someone to climb with!

Just like your client's challenge of where to start, you are faced with a similar question of what views of health, wellness, growth and development to draw upon in your work as a coach. Here is one methodology to consider.

Coaching for Strategic Lifestyle Change

Choosing Strategic	Living Lifestyle	Loving Interpersonal	Being Intrapersonal
Strategic Thinking	Environment	Love or Fear	Internal Aspects
Strategizing	Breathing	Conflict Skills	Belief Systems
Conscious Living	Moving	Conflict Resolution	Cognitive Thinking
Awareness	Eating	Communication Skills	Spiritual
Delegation	Centering &Relaxation	Connectedness	Self Talk
Values	Yoga	Support	Gremlin Fighting
Goal Clarification	Tai Chi	Inclusion	Self Worth
Priorities	Meditation	Camaradarie	Self Esteem
Thrive Not Survive	Exercise	Family	Self Expression
Re-owning		History	Play
Urgent/Important			
Travel Time			

TABLE 9.1

Choosing: Coaching the Strategic Aspects of Life

Strategic Thinking	True Priorities
Strategizing	Urgent / Important
Conscious Living	Thrive, don't just survive
Delegation	Re-owning
Values and Goals Clarification	

Our big brains seem to often be a liability when we believe that our intellect is the only guide to follow. However, effective use of that huge cerebral cortex that has allowed us, as a species, to adapt and survive, even thrive. We all problem solve, integrate, synthesize and process information. We deduce, assume, presume, construe, infer and conclude many things. We are, at times, our own worst enemy and our own savior. Like many human gifts the intellect seem to shine when we engage with others in our quest.

Coaching is an expedient process that allows our clients to find what will be most advantageous in less time. Through engaging with your client in strategic thinking you can help them to actualize and put into operation the goals they are pursuing. We have rightly emphasized motivation throughout this book. An equal number of failed attempts to reach the summit of the mountain can be attributed to poor planning and execution. Strategic thinking with your client is the practical, roll-up-the-sleeves part of coaching that is really fun! Your client's energy and excitement will be a boon to their progress and good strategic thinking can stimulate it.

Goal Selection Based On True Priorities

The order to the steps your client uses to move towards a wellness lifestyle may not seem so important, but they are. Certainly someone can improve their diet, gain sleep and develop and stick to an exercise routine at the same time. For most people the wellness to do list can be imposing and even impractical. People have so many good wellness ideas and intentions and so little time.

Priorities can guide us in our selection of where to put our energy (time, attention, effort, resources). However, not everything can be a priority. You might say that part of the definition of a priority is that there aren't very many of them! So what are our true priorities? They are the ones rooted most deeply into our core beliefs and values. Our true priorities serve us best when they are centered in compassion for others and for self as well. Coaching can help us to distinguish what really is important to us, and how urgent it really is.

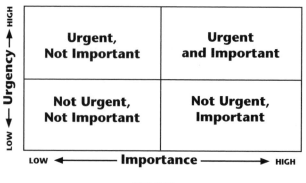

FIGURE 9.1

Help your client process the items from their wellness to do list through this matrix. You will see that not everything is of high importance and/or urgent. If your client feels like everything belongs at the highest level, it's time to spend more processing time with their coach!

Important

A good hard look at what really IS important, what truly matters to us will sometimes open our eyes. Coach your client to help them clarify their values. Help them to seek alignment with their own values. Have your client ask himself or herself, "How does this serve me, others and the world around me?" "Is this an expression of who I am?" "Am I being true to myself?" Help them experiment with perspective by asking themselves "How will this serve me in the future or in the long run?"

Urgent

Over the years I've found myself advising clients to "never make a decision just to relieve anxiety." If you are worried and highly anxious about something, deal with the anxiety first. Relax and center yourself first. Work on the feelings first rather than seeking a quick fix from a not-so-well-thought-out decision.

Conscious Living

As mentioned before, part of your job as a wellness coach is to remind people that they have choices! Good strategies are well thought out and consciously deployed and employed. When your client seems to encounter obstacles help them distinguish between real circumstance and ones of their own making. Obstacles of real circumstance can usually be seen as challenges to be overcome and a way can usually be found. If not, it's time to go back to the drawing board and rework the goal.

Obstacles of our own making can be more feeling based. If your client says, "Well, I can't go and do my exercise workout there because I don't know anybody." help them examine this conclusion. Could they find a place to workout where they know people? They may begin to see how they are creating ways of holding themselves back and may need to talk about their fears of rejection, and their feelings of isolation. As an effective coach we need to be able to address both partners, the head and the heart.

Drawing Distinctions

When we use the urgent/important matrix we are drawing distinctions. Distinctions are one of the primary tools in the masterful coach's tool box. When clients do not distinguish between urgent and important they feel constantly overwhelmed. As a coach you can ask powerful questions to challenge your client to explore different perspectives on key concepts that seem to be guiding their lives and determining the course of immediate action. I've always found that this is where many of the "Ah-ha!" moments are for my clients. The insights they gain from examining distinctions open up their options and often correct the course they are on.

Looking at such distinctions as: can't vs. won't; hope vs. faith; adjusting to vs. tolerating; and surrender vs. accept, etc., can spawn stimulating and insightful explorations. You can either suggest to your client the distinction to be drawn, "Do you believe this is a matter of wishing and hoping or of having faith?" Or, you can ask them to create and draw the distinction themselves, "What are you really looking at here? Is it a matter of trying harder, or is it something else?"

Thomas Leonard was extremely fond of this process and made it a foundational technique of the coaching he taught. His fascination with words and lists drew him to develop a *Distinctionary of Concepts* that serves as a great resource for coaches. (http://coachville.com/tl/distinctionary//dix.html)

Delegation

Most every book on success implores us to delegate, delegate, delegate. It is another classic "Sure, I know to do it, but I don't." scenario. A client who wants to live a high-level wellness lifestyle will always be challenged with finding the time for it and with managing stress. Delegation sounds like a simple and fantastic solution. Where possible just hand some of the work to others who can help. Wow! Sounds great! However even where the work force of helpers is actually there, all too often delegation is not employed. My clients have often felt overwhelmed by work at home or in the workplace when able-bodied spouses, children, co-workers and employees were available to help.

Coach your client around delegation by having them ask themselves these powerful questions:

1. WHO do I actually (truly) have available to delegate to?

2. Have I TRAINED them to receive delegation from me or not?

3. Do I TRUST their competency? (Have I trained them to be competent?)

4. Do I make delegation PERSONAL when it really isn't?

5. What am I AFRAID of when I consider delegating?

It is astonishing sometimes how emotionally laden delegation can be. If it was a simple, logical and practical decision to delegate would be easier and occur more often. I've even had clients who own their own business reluctant to delegate to employees the very tasks they were hired to do! To my client it felt like their employee who was hired to file the office files was doing a personal favor instead of her job.

Finding the way out of this emotional mine field is difficult. Together you and your client can explore delegation, set up experiments and then explore the results, both in terms of practical satisfaction, and the emotional component. Effective delegation creates the freedom to be more efficient and effective at work and at home creating the freedom to include more self-care and wellness in life.

Conscious Calendarizing

As simple as it sounds, urge your clients to be more realistic about time. The pace of life in the modern (especially urban) world has accelerated creating a time famine. When I presented about wellness and stress management in Thailand, I was astonished to hear urban Thais describing an exhausting lifestyle filled with traffic jams, excessive office work loads, and not enough time! Even in a land famous for massage and meditation, people were not using what was available to them and were experiencing many of the same stressors and stress related disorders we see elsewhere in the world.

Coach your client to be more conscious about time by:

1. Exploring their experience and perception of time.

2. Experimenting with putting everything on a calendar.

Make calendarizing a new term. Not everyone has an accountant-like affinity for writing everything down, so you will have to strategize with your client and develop custom-made ways that will work for her or him. Experiment with putting both work and wellness self-care items on the calendar. Help your client to recognize and operate again from true priorities, acknowledging the paramount importance of their own health.

Avoiding Action Evaporation

"Life happens!" Ah yes, the universal excuse (and sometimes very legitimate one) for not getting committed actions completed, especially wellness/self-care items. Life does indeed happen, so how do you help your client regroup when it does? An effective method I've developed to help avoid time evaporation is the following:

1. Calendarize as much as possible; make commitments to take action and designate the time to do so. Set up a designated start and stop day for the week (demarcating the calendar week).

2. When a unit of time (an hour, half-hour, etc.) set aside for a committed action is passed over (not used for that purpose) take note of it.

3. Reassign that unit of time to another time within that same calendar week.

4. Make a commitment to completing this committed action within the same week. Do not allow it to escape the week and evaporate.

5. Keep track of any unit of time that is not used for committed action completion in the week and put it onto a list entitled "Self-deception Units" or "B.S. Units."

6. Set up coaching accountability and coaching agreements around all of this.

The possibilities for coaching the strategic aspects of living a healthy lifestyle are only as limited as you think they are! Have fun exploring and experimenting with your clients. Co-creating strategies that really work are some of the fun parts of wellness coaching.

Living: Lifestyle Improvement Coaching

Nourishing/Moving /Centering	Centering & Relaxation Methods
Environment	Yoga
Breathing	Tai Chi
Moving	Meditation
Eating	

The second realm in our view of wellness is what we refer to as living. Coaching for lifestyle improvement involves many things, but here we will focus on some of the actions that are practical and affect our health directly. Let us bring some structure to our wellness coaching here by looking at how we nourish, move and center ourselves.

Environmental Nourishment

The environment around us either nourishes us or denies us nourishment. We are nourished by clean air, clean water, nutritious food, and safe surroundings where energy can flow into us and out of us efficiently. An important and often overlooked part of living a wellness lifestyle is conscious awareness of our environment. What aspects of our environment can we affect directly (e.g. using less air conditioning, learning and using Feng Shui principles), and what can we affect in concert with others (e.g. help establish a local bike trail, lobby for safer lighting in our neighborhood, support candidates devoted to clean environments)? What aspects are we unable to control, short of re-locating?

In the Wheel of Life illustrated earlier in this book a person is asked to visually show their level of satisfaction with their environment. They are invited to demonstrate how satisfied they are with where they live and work and how their wellness options are limited or enhanced by where they live.

Some communities have abundant resources for safe outdoor exercise such as walking and bicycle trails, tennis and basketball courts, swimming pools or clean lakes. Some communities do not. The city I live by today is a dreamscape of outdoor and public recreation options: parks, playgrounds, public swimming pools, an ice arena, and an extensive network of bicycle trails and wide streets that include bicycle lanes. My old hometown has zero parks, tennis courts, public paths or trails, its streets and highways have virtually no room for bicycles, and this was one of the reasons I moved. Your client may benefit from looking at their community and the area where they live with a critical eye for built-in wellness recreation resources, or the lack thereof.

As you coach your client on various areas of focus you will undoubtedly encounter environmental aspects to their wellness goals. They may feel fortunate to have a lot of opportunities easily available. They may feel blocked from being as healthy as they would like to be because of lack of opportunity. As they become more and more conscious of their own way of living and how it affects their health, they may begin to realize the toll that factors such as noise, crowding, polluted air (both indoor and outdoor), and stressful long commutes are taking. Their sense of connectedness to the natural world is also important to examine. Time in nature refreshes mind, body and spirit. A sense of perspective is regained and our experience of ourselves is deepened. A U.S. Forest Service study confirmed that one third of the visitors to National Forests went there primarily for spiritual purposes. Your wellness coaching may involve more strategizing with your client on how they can make the best use of their environment to get the nourishment they need.

When communities of people have access to a safe place to get out and move they are healthier. A great resource for looking at this is the work of Dr. James Sallis and the Active Living Research Foundation (???) –INDICATE RESOURCE REFERRENCE - Their research showed that communities with poor health statistics were able to vastly improve indicators of their health once safe places to walk/exercise were established. Wellness professionals and public parks and planning agencies can make a big difference working together.

Nourishing The Body/Mind

The body is nourished by air, water and earth. Air is often considered the breath of life and Prana, the life force that we breathe in. Air quality is the first level of awareness and it is important to improve it. How we breathe is the next. The more anxious we are the more our breath is short and shallow. Conscious awareness of our breath allows us to relax and to take in more of what we need to nourish ourselves. There are many ways in which our clients can benefit from learning breathing techniques and methodologies. Reclaiming our breath (lung capacity) after surgery and/or illness is often a very important part of the recovery process.

Water nourishes us on a deeply cellular level. It flushes toxins away and restores homeostasis in our bodies. The effects of dehydration, either chronic or acute, can be truly amazing, ranging from kidney disorders to temporary mental derangement. Clearly we need good clean water and plenty of it.

Our wellness clients can benefit from good health information about the purity of the water they are drinking. Many municipal water sources are questionable in quality and when tested by a reputable firm show unwanted toxic content. Be safe by being aware. Most effective weight loss programs also find that there is greater success when people adequately hydrate their bodies.

The earth nourishes us in many ways, but of course it is the source of the food we eat . . . all of it! Healthy food starts at the source with clean soil and clean water, with limited or no chemicals. As I once heard the late Paul Knoop, an inspirational Audubon Society naturalist, say "Absolutely everything comes from a green leaf." Once the quality of our food is established the great quandary and great debate begins over what to choose to eat!

We come back to the word nourishing. Does the food I am eating truly nourish me? Is it what I (as a unique human being) need? Food is far more than calories of energy to burn. It supplies us with chemicals that our bodies need on many levels. Some of these we are aware of and some we are only beginning to discover. Whole foods supply us with both our known and unknown requirements, as long as we are eating a rich variety of good quality foods. Wellness coaching clients may have any of a number of unique food considerations. We can encourage them to factor in (perhaps with the help of professional nutritionists) their body composition goals, metabolic rate, allergies and sensitivities, hormones, and the requirements that their unique health challenges may impose.

As stated in our earlier section on motivation, eating is a behavior. It is a topic that only begins with health information. Most of our clients know basically what and how much they need to eat to be well (whether they are doing it or not). Wellness coaching regarding nourishing the body is not just straightforward hard science. It crosses over quickly into the so-called soft sciences of psychology, sociology and even anthropology. Eating behavior is multi-causal. It is a result of emotions, self-beliefs, culture and sub-culture. Media, peer health norms, traditions and accessibility influence our eating behavior. The job of a coach is to help our client become conscious of their eating behavior and to develop effective ways of improving it.

As tempting as it is to teach and preach about the benefits of making certain food choices, and eating in certain ways, we come back once again to coaching. Here we challenge our clients to become more and more conscious of their eating behavior. Conscious awareness is a very powerful antidote to the thoughtless eating behavior that operates on automatic pilot and steers us into self-defeating choices. Tracking techniques such as conscious meal planning and recording can help tremendously. Becoming our client's ally and support system in whatever healthy eating plan they choose and develop for themselves is one of the best ways we can serve them. The accountability methods of coaching can help your clients be consistent enough for them to experience success.

Keep yourself informed and aware of current information about all the diets that become popular. We see diets come and go, some achieving acceptance as healthy and beneficial, and others discredited and eventually abandoned. This is truly the arena of "If it sounds too good to be true, it probably is!" Encourage your client to check into the validity of a particular diet they are attracted to. Become familiar with qualified nutritionists in your area and refer to them often.

Moving the Body/Mind

The only way to make sense out of change is to plunge into it, move with it, and join the dance.

—Alan Watts

We are designed to move. When there is flow, there is life. The enemy of health is blockage of flow. That blockage can be either outside of us or inside. An external blockage will be something we tend to strain against. If we do not succeed in moving the blockage we may get discouraged, give up or possibly find a way to adapt. Internal blockage may hinder our effort to move. Emotional paralysis, like its physical counterpart, is truly tragic. One often leads to the other.

Whether we are looking at ancient Taoist texts, manuals for Chinese medicine, or John Travis's energy flow model for wellness, we are talking about flow. Unimpeded flow of energy is often expressed in movement of one type or another. The result of such flow is a state of good health . . . wellness!

Challenging all of our clients (and ourselves!) is a world where conditions have increased the sedentary factor in life. The more sedentary we are the more sedated we become. Working with data all day, driving and riding almost everywhere, the rise of sedentary recreation, all combine to numb us into a lack of awareness and a loss of health. We now recognize sedentary lifestyles as a major health risk.

Wellness is often mistakenly equated solely with our level of physical fitness. Think of a wellness program and you picture a gym type of setting with people working out. For some of our clients the word exercise is loaded with negative memories and connotations. Yet, most wellness-coaching clients know that being more physically fit is indeed a vital part of living well. Most of our clients want the results of exercise yet it may not be a part of their lives. Like dieting, the world of exercise often means memories of failed attempts at establishing plans that did not work. It may even bring up painful memories of gym classes and social situations where being less than a perfect athlete led to embarrassment and shame. This is where the coach approach is so critical to success.

We start with the mindset shift from the prescriptive to the coach-like. Instead of coming up with a person's ideal workout routine or having them buy into a specific exercise method, we coach, we provide an ally for them to explore their options and create experiments where we will provide continuous support. We may not be out there physically moving on the bike path or the swimming pool, with them, but through our coaching process of exploration, support and accountability we are with them.

Just as in the area of nutrition, you need to be a coach, not the expert. Again you join the client in the exploration of creating and/or choosing a wellness plan that works for them. Expanding the concept to movement makes it easier for the client to see ways to improve in this area. Much of your work regarding this area will be around motivation and all the excuses not to exercise.

You may not want to talk about exercise at all. Encourage your client to simply increase movement in their lives. Make a fun project out of helping them discover everyday ways that they can move more. Conscious awareness is our ally here. One client of mine had a profound revelation when she realized that she had engineered her life to minimize movement. She used this realization to flip her thinking around into more and more creative ways to move more in everyday life. This progressed from parking further away, taking the stairs and doing more errands on foot herself, to actually signing up for a vigorous dance class and even dusting off her long-abandoned treadmill and using it!

As a wellness coach you will help your client:

- Explore their beliefs, myths, self-defeating behaviors and patterns around movement/exercise (the internal blockages).

- Strategize practical ways to find/create time to exercise.

- Be more realistic and commit to doing less, and at times challenge them to commit to doing more.

- Gain accurate information about ways to exercise.

- Find outside resources (such as fitness trainers, Yoga or Tai Chi teachers).

Just as we stated about the area of eating, the more knowledge of leading wellness information that you have about movement the better. If you are up-to-date in this area you can turn clients on to new methods that might be just right for them to try.

Healthy physical movement includes three major areas:

- Cardio-vascular fitness—endurance

- Strength

- Flexibility

Help your client to find a balance of all three elements. Help them explore their ways of avoidance in one physical movement area and coach them towards balance. (See the Wheel of Physical Satisfaction on page 139.)

A special note. As the baby boom generation ages, we are finding them to be the most physically active of any generation in history. They desire an active life and if they have a history of exercising regularly, may want coaching assistance to adjust to the physical realities of aging. Many runners are now seeking kinder and gentler ways of moving that don't stress the joints as much. Shifting into more balanced movement can help immensely. Flexibility is especially important as we age. Helping your clients explore new ways to stretch the aging muscles will be beneficial. They can try areas that may be new to them, or old passions that were abandoned and now wait to be rediscovered, like dance! Also, we live in a time when the aging joints are being replaced and the client may need your assistance adapting. Urge your clients to get the medical assessments they need and then be their ally in creating and committing to new ways of moving.

The dance is a poem of which each movement is a word.

—Mata Hari

Centered Body — Centered Mind

How we move through life may be just as important as moving itself. Achieving unblocked flow of energy is vital to health. When we describe our lives as being out of balance we are often talking about excessive stress and often much futile effort. What we seek is a centered way to move through life.

You may not be a martial artist, a trained mediator, or a practitioner of Tai Chi. You may not be a trained athlete whose performance depends on how balanced they are on a ski slope or an ice rink. You may not be a professional dancer whose moves reflect what appears to be effortless grace. So you may not be familiar with the term centering.

Be centered. Center yourself. Come from center. Move from center. Return to center. Centering practice. Unless you are watching Kung Fu movies or remember what Obi Wan Kanobi was saying about The Force in Star Wars, you might not hear phrases like this. Yet this concept, once understood and applied, can dramatically improve your life.

You have experienced what I am referring to as being centered and did not even know it. When you made a decision without anxiety, which was true to yourself, that was being centered. When you sank a long putt, a three-point shot, or hit a solid line drive, that was being centered. When you twirled on the dance floor beautifully, carved your best run on a snowboard, or made the perfect cast with your fishing rod that was being centered. You were in the zone. When you found a poem or piece of expressive writing just flowing out of you like liquid, that was experiencing a centered state. When you ended a relationship, not to relieve anxiety or fear, but because you knew, with calm certainty, that it was the best and right thing to do, that too was being centered.

Think of how different your life can be when you realize that being centered is always an option you have in every situation. Think of the effectiveness of decision-making and creativity of effort that can result from operating more from a centered state.

How do we become centered? Instead of it being a magical and elusive state that is hard to recreate, what if centering was a skill that you developed and practiced? What if knowing how to center yourself was accessible information that you could draw upon in conflict, in emergencies, and in opportunities that demand peak performance?

A centered body centers the mind. Centering has a physical aspect to it as well as mental/emotional aspects. They affect each other and you can start in either domain.

Quieting your thoughts will relax your body. Nervous and fearful self-talk can produce muscle tension, increased heart rate, blood pressure, stomach acid production, and more. Quieting the internal chatter and soothing yourself with more positive and calm self-talk, or enhancing it with mental images of tranquil and safe, even idyllic settings has just the opposite effect on the body.

Centering Mind and Body Experience

Physically center yourself by focusing on your breath, changing your posture, lowering your center of gravity and movement, broadening your stance, becoming more in balance. Breathe slower on each breath, and a little deeper. Close your eyes for a moment, perhaps. Sit up straight, or stand with your feet further apart, your knees slightly bent, your weight equally distributed on both feet. As you do this, and breathe in and out slowly and consciously, you'll notice that your mind is slowing down and you are focusing more on the present moment.

Move from center. Place your right index finger in your naval . . . yes, your belly button! Now take your first three fingers of your left hand and place them across your belly right below your right index finger. At that level on your belly where the third finger rests imagine the point that is half-way between your belly and the skin on your back. That spot right in the center of you is what the Chinese call "Tan Tien." The Japanese call it the "Hara" center. Imagine that this is where your body moves from, not up higher somewhere.

Stand like you have just mounted an invisible horse. This is the horse riding stance that you see martial artists assume in martial arts movies and demonstrations. Keep your back relaxed but nice and straight. Look straight ahead. Now flex your knees and shift your weight back and forth from one leg to the other while keeping your feet flat on the ground. Feel very connected to the ground you are standing on. Take small steps with one foot while leaving the other one planted." Move so "Tan Tien" is just floating at the same level all the time.

Experiment with how movement feels in this stance and by moving in this way. Continue to breathe fully and completely. Practice this for five or ten minutes several times a week.

Like the muscular concept of *optimal tonus* what we are looking for here is neither deep relaxation nor rigid tightness. The horse-riding stance is one in which you can feel very solid. Someone who is centered in this stance is no push over. It is a stance from which you can move quickly and in which you are very flexible. No energy is being wasted on muscles that are not involved in holding the posture itself. Those unused muscles are at rest. Movement comes from your true center.

The next time you need to make an important decision, or deal with a challenging situation, just adopt this stance. When the others around you stop laughing the conflict will be over. Yes, I am kidding! Getting yourself centered physically can really help though, so try less obvious methods like the following.

Centering In Action

Breathe. A good, long, slow, deep breath can do wonders. It cues your mind to come out of a tendency toward overwhelm or panic, and allows you to take in more immediate information about the situation. Sit up or stand very straight, with your feet firmly planted on the floor or ground.

Now the mental part! Think of this "Tan Tien" center in your body and adopt the ancient Samurai notion of expect nothing, be prepared for anything. Be aware of everything around you where you are, right here and right now in the present moment. Let the past and future evaporate. Focus on the present.

Bring your thoughts to an observation of the present situation without letting your past biases influence it. Take what the moment brings you without judgment. Then from that calm, centered place make a distinction between your choices, based on the values that are true to you.

Coach a Centered Life

There are real benefits to engaging in a formally trained centering practice. The tremendous rise in popularity of meditation, mindfulness, Yoga and Tai Chi worldwide is evidence of this. Your coaching clients may find activities like this to be an ideal complement to the more vigorous fitness activities they engage in.

There are activities that we can participate in to deeply relax, bringing out the psycho-physiological response we call the relaxation response (parasympathetic nervous system arousal) such as relaxation training, biofeedback, meditation, self-hypnosis, etc. There are also ways that we relax that are less intense but very important to us. Likewise there are probably favorite activities that your clients engage in that produce in them, to some degree, this experience of centering. They are usually activities that are very healthy, that give them perspective, that refresh and renew them. They may be as simple as a walk in the park, a hike in someplace a bit wild, throwing pottery, gardening, or just getting together with good friends with no agenda or expectations.

1. Suggest to your client that they create a list of activities of what centers them in their lives.
2. Have them indicate when they last engaged in those activities.
3. Explore their thoughts and feelings about the activity and the lack of it.
4. Explore how ready they are to take some action to do some of the activities that help them center again.
5. Secure a coaching agreement for either preparation or action and include timing.

Loving: Coaching the Interpersonal Aspects of Life

Love or Fear	Community
Conflict Skills	Support
Conflict Resolution	Inclusion
Communication Skills	Camaraderie/Friendship
Connectedness	Play

Coaching sage Thomas Leonard would extol coaches to help their clients to succeed in life by eliminating tolerations and getting their needs met. Some of our most near and dear needs are interpersonal. We all have needs for inclusion and belonging, to nurture and be nurtured. When we look at health statistics it's clear we just don't do well alone. Partnered people live longer and have better health. People with pets do even better!

How connected or isolated our clients are in their lives seems to be a huge determinant not only of their overall health, but their likelihood of success in adopting new lifestyle improving behaviors. As they strive to improve the way they move, eat and manage stress, it all has interpersonal impacts. There is the need for support and for positive peer health norms. This is an opportunity for conflict. Our clients need approval from the people around them—for people to get on board with the changes they are making rather than people who resist their changes.

We certainly train people in how to treat us, not through workshops or seminars, but in our everyday lives. Co-workers may come to expect our client to do all the busy work. What happens when they become more assertive and demand that the busy work be distributed fairly? The experience of re-training others and their response to our client's efforts may become an important part of coaching.

What happens when our client decides to reduce and eventually eliminate red meat from the family dinner menu? What happens in a partnership or family when a new diagnosis means our client radically alters the way they eat? Wellness becomes a very interpersonal issue.

Coach for Connectedness

During the coaching process you become an ally for your client, accompanying them on their wellness journey. A lot of the effectiveness of coaching seems linked to the support our client receives from their relationship with us. What's next? Not only will we not be coaching them forever, we are not physically around after our brief meeting each week. Who picks up the slack, both now, and in the future?

Coaching the building and bolstering of support systems may be the single most important work we do with our clients. Introduce the concept of connectedness and community early in your coaching. Check out their current level of isolation/connectedness (See The Wellness Mapping 360° Connectedness Scale, Figure 9.2) and the nature and extent of their interpersonal support systems during the foundation session.

There are many sociological factors contributing to the epidemic of loneliness, depression and isolation that we are seeing in the modern world. Robert D. Putnam, in *Bowling Alone: The Collapse and*

Revival of American Community, highlights some of these:

- One in five Americans moves once a year.
- Two in five Americans expect to move in five years.

The CONNECTION SCALE

Explore each statement below and rate (1-5) how true each is for you at this time in your life. Talk with your coach (or a friend) about your answers or write about the experience in your guided wellness journal. Once you rate yourself for each statement add your numbers together to gain your total connectedness score.

1= *Not True*   2= *Hardly ever True*   3= *Sometimes True*   4= *True most of the time*   5 = *True*

Connection to self
1. I enjoy spending time alone. — 1. 2. 3. 4. 5.
2. I have enough time alone. — 1. 2. 3. 4. 5.
3. I am compassionate with myself. — 1. 2. 3. 4. 5.
4. I like who I am as a person. — 1. 2. 3. 4. 5.
5. I like my body. — 1. 2. 3. 4. 5.

Connection to nature and my environment
1. My living space is comfortable and suits me. — 1. 2. 3. 4. 5.
2. I spend quality time in nature. — 1. 2. 3. 4. 5.
3. I have a place I go to for refuge or to recharge. — 1. 2. 3. 4. 5.
4. My workspace is comfortable and suits me. — 1. 2. 3. 4. 5.
5. I know my neighbors. — 1. 2. 3. 4. 5.

Connection to family
1. I have a supportive family. — 1. 2. 3. 4. 5.
2. I enjoy spending time with my family. — 1. 2. 3. 4. 5.
3. I spend enough time with my family. — 1. 2. 3. 4. 5.
4. I feel connected to my family. — 1. 2. 3. 4. 5.
5. I feel a connection to those who came before me. — 1. 2. 3. 4. 5.

Social Connection
1. I spend enough time doing activities I enjoy. — 1. 2. 3. 4. 5.
2. I spend enough time with friends. — 1. 2. 3. 4. 5.
3. I belong to a supportive community. — 1. 2. 3. 4. 5.
4. I have someone I can share most everything with. — 1. 2. 3. 4. 5.
5. I enjoy intimacy. — 1. 2. 3. 4. 5.

Spiritual Connection
1. I feel connected to something greater than myself. — 1. 2. 3. 4. 5.
2. I spend time in a spiritual practice. — 1. 2. 3. 4. 5.
3. I feel a sense of purpose in my life. — 1. 2. 3. 4. 5.
4. I belong to a spiritual group. — 1. 2. 3. 4. 5.
5. I am a spiritual being. — 1. 2. 3. 4. 5.

Connection at work
1. I get along well with my co-workers. — 1. 2. 3. 4. 5.
2. I feel respected in the work I do. — 1. 2. 3. 4. 5.
3. I am part of a team at work. — 1. 2. 3. 4. 5.
4. I have adequate contact with others in the work I do. — 1. 2. 3. 4. 5.
5. My colleagues and I trust one another. — 1. 2. 3. 4. 5.

Total ____

Working With The Connectedness Scale
100 pts – 150 pts = High level of Connectedness – Wonderful, make good use of the support you have
50 pts – 99 pts = Moderate level of Connectedness – OK, talk /write about your satisfaction with the level of support in your life. Consider adding to your Wellness Map
1 pts – 49 pts = Low level of Connectedness – consider adding support systems to your life and your Wellness Map.

Wellness Mapping 360° © Tools for Living Well   *Real Balance Global Wellness Services llc - Copyright 2004*
Reproducible Worksheet Masters are available for purchase on CD ROM from Whole Person Associates, 101 W. 2nd ST., Suite 203, Duluth, MN 55802, 800-247-6789, www.wholeperson.com.

FIGURE 9.2

- In 1950 single person households were less than 10% of the U.S. population; one of every three households created in the 1990s was a single person household.

- There are more single person households—33.6% than there are households of couples with children—33.1%.

- Increasingly, corporate employees work more with data more and less with people.

- More people in the United States are self-employed (which often has an isolating effect) today than at any time since the Industrial Revolution began.

A new study of social isolation (Smith-Lovin, L., McPherson, M., Brashers, M. "Social Isolation in America: Changes in Core Discussion Networks Over Two Decades" *American Sociological Review* 71:3, 2006) concluded that in 1985 the average American had three people in his or her closest intimate circles—people in whom they confide matters important to them. In 2004 the number has dropped to only *one*! They also found that 25% of Americans have no one to confide in at all. As a wellness coach, you may have a profound role in helping your clients build social support systems and to become less isolated.

You may be your client's first experience with a trusted ally. A psychiatrist I used to work with would often say that a client needed a "corrective emotional experience." What she often meant was that by trusting a counselor (or in this case, a coach) the client learned to trust. Do not underestimate the power of the coaching relationship. Sometimes the anchor our clients have with us allows them to feel safe enough to take the risk and reach out to others.

As you coach, continually check in with your client about the involvement of others in their wellness goals. Help them explore the fears that may hold them back from seeking more support. Are they ashamed to need help? Do they see asking for support as a sign of weakness? Are they afraid of rejection? Does it go against the norms of their family, culture, or sub-culture to invite someone in or to change specific behavior? Have they been refused support before? Do they truly have non-supportive people surrounding them, or are they too isolated?

227

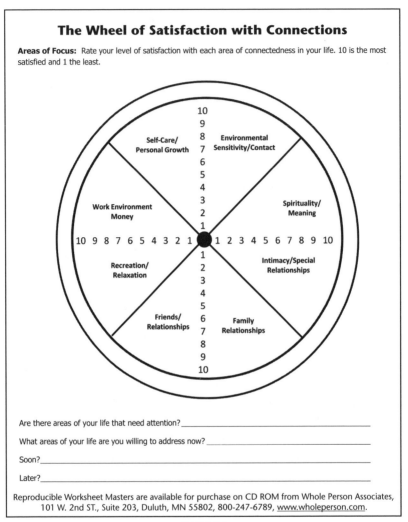

FIGURE 9.3

Help your client to see securing support as a key to maintaining lifestyle improvements they have made. At the close of your coaching relationship it is most likely that the change process and the continued adoption of new health behaviors will not be complete. Who can help them follow through what Prochaska calls the sixth stage of change—termination—to give the new behavior the time needed to habituate?

Coach for Community and Support

Keeping in mind the findings of Smith-Lovin, McPherson and Brashears (pgs. 180, 181), we should consider the following points as we coach our clients.

- Build sources of support right into the Wellness Plan.
- As new action steps emerge see if there is a connectedness component to be included.
- Ask permission to explore your clients fears about connection with others. Explore the value they see (or don't see) in community.
- Explore how their thinking (and inner-critic activity) affects their efforts at connecting with others.
- For the client who needs to develop more sources of support, make it one of their Areas of Focus in their Wellness Plan. Work together to create goals and action steps that make increasing connectedness a very conscious effort.
- Strategize with your client how they can build greater community into their life.
- As the termination of coaching approaches, increase the emphasis on building support systems that will continue to help the client to grow and maintain the success they've achieved.

No one is to be called an enemy, all are your benefactors,
and no one does you harm. You have no enemy except
yourselves.
— **St. Francis of Assisi**

Being: Coaching the Intrapersonal Self

The Internal Aspects	Meaning—Purpose
Belief System Cognitive—Spiritual	Self-worth—Self-esteem
Self-talk	Self-expression
Gremlin Fighting	Play

It is not the mountain we conquer but ourselves.

— **Edmund Hillary**

I'm a long-time fan of Johnny Hart's comic strip "B.C." A recurrent theme in the strip is to have a character climb a steep mountain peak and ask the wise old man with the long white beard what the meaning of life really is. There is always some satirical comment that makes us laugh. The humor always hits home because we are laughing at ourselves. Don't we spend way too much time and energy in our lives looking for the answers outside of ourselves? Finding meaning, living a life on purpose, and understanding our reality is like a perpetual quest. Is that the real Holy Grail that everyone from the creators of the Monty Python movies, to author Tom Brown (*The Davinci Code*), to philosophers and Popes all talk about?

> *The Creator gathered all of Creation and said, "I want to hide something from the humans until they are ready for it. It is the realization that they create their own reality." The eagle said, "Give it to me, I will take it to the moon." The Creator said, "No. One day they will go there and find it." The salmon said, "I will bury it on the bottom of the ocean." "No. They will go there too." The buffalo said, "I will bury it on the Great Plains." The Creator said, "They will cut into the skin of the Earth and find it even there."*
>
> *Grandmother Mole, who lives in the breast of Mother Earth, and who has no physical eyes but sees with spiritual eyes, said, "Put it inside of them." And the Creator said, "It is done."*
>
> **—A Sioux Creation Myth**

Wellness author Don Ardell has long contended that we will achieve better results in our efforts to help people accomplish lasting lifestyle change if we tie it in to the quest for meaning in life. He proposes that we encourage people to think of meaning, purpose and happiness in four structured parts:

1. The ground floor of meaning is subsistence/safety and security seeking. For most this is the orientation that gets attention throughout life. It means your job, career, and all that connects with securing the means to get by, preferably in a little style and comfort.

2. Meaning at the leisure level. This entails some concern

for living wisely, agreeably and well (a phrase attributed to John Maynard Keynes). Maslow called this level belongingness in his famous hierarchy of needs construct.

3. Meaning found in the development, refinement and expression of talents, gifts and uniqueness. It entails self-fulfillment and earned self-esteem.

4. Meaning from reaching out and being of service. This could entail meeting needs of others, or the pursuit of knowledge for the betterment of society.

Ardell, D (2003) HENROD conference April 24, 2003. Newark, Delaware @ Used by permission.

The internal aspects of wellness seem like a limitless universe of topics, ideas, concepts, wonderings, and wanderings. Again, how do we help our clients to tread in this territory without getting lost in space? I think Ardell's four structures ground the topic of meaning very practically. While you may never have a conversation directly about "the meaning of life" with your client (perhaps those are best left for spiritual retreats, campfires and starlit nights), you can usually tell when a client has work to do in this realm.

We often see it in a lack of motivation or a real inconsistency in motivation. There is a lack or ambivalence of energy to take action. Without meaning and purpose we see those that Thoreau wrote about when he said, "Most men lead lives of quiet desperation." It is really living a life lacking in vision. It is wandering through life, even with a map and a compass, but nowhere to go. You need a map of your own design, not one someone assigned to you. You need your own internal compass and the decision of a destination, above all else, needs to be yours. You are the author of our own life story, and the only true authority on your life.

Much of what we have looked at in this book has been about the internal aspects of wellness. The work on belief systems, thought patterns, self-perceptions, intrinsic and extrinsic motivation, gremlin fighting and more, all contribute to our way of approaching the world and set up what works for us and against us as we seek to give expression to our growth. As you coach your clients you will draw upon this myriad of information from many sources as well as all you have learned in your life about human behavior.

Again and again you will see how the way a person feels about themselves, and what they continually say to themselves about themselves will be a huge determinant of their lifestyle behavior and consequently, of their health. Focusing on self-esteem, self-worth, identity and self-concept are not endeavors necessarily requiring advanced degrees in psychoanalysis. Instead, bring these concepts down to earth with your clients. Put legs under them. Use your coaching skills. Listen deeply. Say what is.

- Let your client know what you are observing, and feed it back to them without judgment. "I see that each time we talk about the goal you said you wanted to work on this week, you change the subject."

- Ask powerful questions. "So, what would happen if you did step forward and ask for what you really want?" Remember that the least powerful question you can ask is "Why?"

- Encourage your client to grant themselves greater permission for self-care, and creative self-expression. Explore what this would actually look like in their life. Help them create experiments around these themes. As they engage more in these two areas, progress will emerge in the way they feel about themselves. As we have said earlier, self-esteem and motivation for change are intimately connected.

A client of mine was a profitable business owner who usually did an excellent job of managing his investments and running his busy agency. Part of what made him so successful was that he truly valued balance. He applied the principle of balance to the way he spread his money around and the way he lived his personal life as well. One of the things he realized as being vital to not only his health and well being, but to his business success as well, was creative self-expression.

My client knew from experience, that when he denied himself his outlets for creative self-expression he felt more stressed, anxious and less confident. He knew that he was far less creative in his work and that his customers were not as attracted to him and to doing more business with him. When he devoted adequate time to his pursuit of creative photography and developed his skills as a potter, then life, health, and business all were better.

Creative self-expression became a primary focus of our coaching and for several months he looked to coaching to help him be accountable to himself in this area. Even when life and work's busy-ness seemed far too pressing, he found value in the coaching process as it helped him center himself more and express himself creatively.

Coaching for Connectedness On the Intrapersonal Level

One Sunday in my teen-age youth, I experienced a profound sermon that was really about connectedness. The minister, who at the time was probably using terms like sin and unforgivable, was actually talking about how the worst state of being a person could be in was that of complete disconnection from their spirituality. I remember being deeply impacted by that message. It rang true for me, and still does.

Our sense of meaning and purpose actually connects us to all the rest of life. The expression of our true self grounds us in the world. How aware we are of our experience is an indication of our connection to all that is within and without. Are we in harmony with all that is around us and inside us? When that harmony is broken, and it will be, how do we regain it quickly? What is your harmony recovery time?

When we enter the realm of the spiritual the coach always completely respects the spiritual and religious traditions and values of our clients. This exploration, like all of coaching, is client-centered and client-driven. For some of our clients going deeper into connection is about connecting with something greater than themselves or even the world around them. It can be a profound source of strength and support for our clients to draw upon when they feel that their spiritual resource (their God, etc.) is right in there with them. Their spiritual community (Church, Synagogue, Mosque, Temple, etc.) may be a tremendous source of support. Your client may select this as an area to work on in coaching so they can make better use of this resource.

Wellness coaching clients thrive on self-awareness and connectedness. We usually think of connectedness as being equivalent to the experience of social support. We may even take a more ecological focus and talk about our connection to the natural world. There is an internal connectedness that our clients benefit from cultivating as well. How can we help them to turn this soil?

Wherever you are, whatever you do, you can always come back to this marvelous sense of stillness, the feeling of yourself, very, very much here. This is your reference point: this is your stability. This is your life force that gives you balance. This is your home you carry around with you wherever you are. This is your powerhouse, your reservoir, your endless inexhaustible resource . . .

—**Al Huang**
Embrace Tiger, Return to Mountain—the Essence of T'ai Chi,
speaking about being centered

Internal connectedness is much more possible when we slow down the pace of our lives, if only temporarily. It is more possible when we are not distracting ourselves from our own experience of the present moment. When we coach for intrinsic motivation we have our clients notice more. We have them notice what they are aware of in their own bodies as they move and exercise. We help them discover the intrinsic rewards in the activity itself, and in doing so, discover the joy as well.

When we ask powerful questions for our clients to reflect upon their experience in the present moment (yes even in the present moment of the coaching appointment), we are helping them to connect with their experience. When we help our clients eliminate clutter from their lives we are helping them reduce distraction so they can focus on the here and now. Help your client discover ways to bring him or herself into the present moment.

Connection to self, to source, to the oneness that we all seek in our own way, is a natural state. It is mostly about removing the things – the behaviors that get in the way. We simply have to get out of our own way. Restoring that natural state of connection may be where some of our best wellness work lies.

Trust the river, but keep the paddle in your hands

Life is like a river, that flows along infinitely. We do not control where the river goes. We do not control the flow of the river, not its crashing rapids nor its quiet still pools. We don't know where the fork on the left goes, or the fork on the right.

We are not driftwood. We are not helplessly being pushed down the river by the current, smashing into the rocks, or stuck in circling eddies.

It is like we are in a canoe, with a paddle in our hands. Sitting high in our seat, our eyes wide open, looking ahead we scan for signs of white water. Our ears alert, we listen for the roar of rapids and waterfalls.

We decide whether to take the fork to the left or the one to the right and we decide whether to run the rapids, or to put ashore and portage around, putting our craft back in the water when it is safe.

Going with the flow of the river we learn to navigate with the current, not against it.

We learn to trust the river, but remember the paddle in our hands. We remember the power of choice we have and know that we did not create the river, but we choose how to live with what it brings us.

Chapter 10

Health and Medical Coaching —Coaching People with Health Challenges

It is natural to resist change—for better or worse. This resistance to change is called homeostasis . . . your body has billions of feedback loops that keep your physiological functions within a narrow, normal equilibrium. And it's a good thing, or you might die . . . The same is true on the emotional and spiritual levels. We tend not to question our beliefs, our perceptions, and our patterns of behavior, even when they are causing problems for us.
The same homeostasis that protects us from change also makes it more difficult for us to transform even when it's in our best interest to do so.

—**Dean Ornish, M.D.,** *Eat More, Weigh Less*

Facing the Health Challenge

Health challenges can take on many forms. We are all faced with the challenge of living well in a world that doesn't always support healthy lifestyle choices. There are times in our lives, however, when the challenge might be much greater. The news of a close relative dying of a genetically linked disease, or a diagnosis of heart disease, cancer, diabetes, osteoporosis or arthritis, just to name a few, really changes people's lives. How we speak of and view these health challenges is important right from the start.

In coaching vernacular problems are translated into challenges. We are not always doomed by our problems, conditions, and diagnoses. It is extremely easy to lose hope and feel victimized by a lab result if we take such news as a final condemnation. Instead, we can shift our mindset and view the problem as a challenge that we must face. Then the possibility of meeting and overcoming the challenge and emerging as a stronger, deeper person becomes possible.

Speaking of a cancer diagnosis as a challenge is not to diminish its seriousness. We had better take it seriously! We know, however, that the people who face their fears and their diagnosis tap into their will to live and be well. When they don't have to do it alone, they often conquer more than just their own fears. A challenge engages a person to do what they can, and then do more. As a coach you have the honor of being a person's ally through this process.

Where Do You Fit In? Coaching and Coaching Skills

For many of you who are attracted to wellness coaching, people who have health challenges are not new, you work with them all the time. As a medical professional you continuously face the challenge when working with your patients: when to stay focused on the treatment methodology and when to recognize that what you are dealing with has crossed over into the world of behavior.

For medical professionals, using the mindset shift to coaching is a huge advantage when addressing behavioral issues. The coaching mindset coupled with coaching skills allows you to support people as they change their lifestyle behavior. As we have said frequently in this book, most wellness and medical personnel discover that just telling people what to do seldom works. Whether you plan to become a full time wellness coach or are a medical professional, training in coaching skills and the recognition of the coaching mindset will serve you and your clients/patients well. For the healthcare worker already inside the medical system coaching skills can transform the way you do one-on-one work. For the wellness coach seeking entry into the system it is a matter of finding forward thinking programs.

When it comes to working with people with health challenges, some coaching students raise concerns about how competent they could be to work with this population. If their background is anything but a nurse or medical treatment professional, they wonder if it is okay to enter into coaching someone with a chronic illness, etc. Whether you call it wellness coaching or health coaching, the reality is that in most cases the vast majority of clients we work with already have some kind of diagnosed medical condition. It may be hypertension, hyperlipidemia or an elevated blood sugar level, or the client may already be dealing with heart disease, diabetes or some other life-threatening illness.

When coaches stick to coaching, and don't stray beyond their "scope of practice" working with clients with medical conditions is not a problem. The coach from a non-medical background does not have to have a treatment-level of knowledge about an illness. They can certainly do better coaching if they acquire a knowledge of their client's illness/challenges that allows them to speak with their client effectively. At this time there is no evidence that a person with a medical background makes a better coach. One large company that provides wellness coaching for clients with diabetes and heart disease actually avoids hiring coaches with a medical background. They find that these coaches do not have to be retrained to make the coaching mindset shift and they stick to coaching, not diagnosing and treating.

To serve your clients the best, and for your own protection, insist that anyone you coach who does have a medical condition be under current and active medical treatment for that condition. Refuse to coach the prospective client who will not agree with this.

Coaching People with Health Challenges

A careful examination of Travis's Wellness/Illness Continuum reveals that the work of wellness begins long before a person becomes ill. Preventing the onset of detectable disease is always preferable. When treatment is needed, the work of wellness and the wellness coach is most beneficial when it engages a person early in the treatment process, either as soon as an issue has been identified through a Health Risk Assessment or early in treatment. The ideal is a scenario where the coach supports a person's behavioral compliance with treatment and the enhancement of the body/mind's own systems for

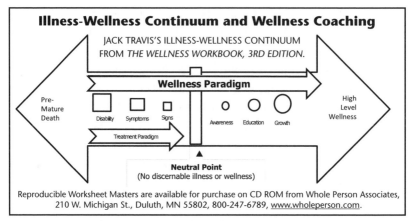

FIGURE 10.1

healing through the practice of a healthy lifestyle. This speeds and insures greater probability of treatment success and reduces present or possible risk factors. In addition to the internal healing process, it is important for medical professionals engaged in the treatment methodology to work hand-in-hand with behavioral change specialists to bring an ill person back to the midpoint, the point of no discernable illness. The Wellness Coach can be a vital part of this process.

Coaching for Prevention After a Warning Signal

There is an old saying that "heart attacks usually don't just happen overnight." Progressive diseases such as coronary artery disease are slow in development and sometimes go unnoticed until a serious condition has developed. Often though, for many health challenges there are some warnings that show up earlier.

In my stress management seminars I would often have people imagine driving a car down a highway and have them look at the gauges on the car's dashboard. I would ask them to imagine seeing the temperature gauge cause the red warning light to come on, and then ask them "What do you do?" Most people would say, "Pull off the road and check it out!" but others would humorously, but honestly admit they would just keep on driving! Unfortunately this same approach applies when it comes to the red lights on our own control panel of health.

In working for years with people with stress-related disorders I saw that stress had a way of sending its warning messages. If the low-level messages like insomnia and headache were ignored, then stress had a way of upping the ante, that is, increasing the stakes. The next round of warnings could be much more serious and include things like the onset of symptoms of physical conditions and disease processes such as gastrointestinal disorders, debilitating headaches or high blood pressure.

Many health conditions respond well to lifestyle improvement alone, if the lifestyle changes are early and sufficient enough. The role of wellness coaching in this level of prevention can be very valuable. Wellness programs have long sought to identify people who are at risk earlier and earlier. Once identified, there is something that wellness coaches can actually do to change clients' risks beyond just giving them more information. You can give the client an ally to help insure that they make the lifestyle changes that will address the health warning they have received. In many ways wellness coaching helps a person make use of the information they have and what they know.

Target potential clients who are in this early warning category. If they are ready to take their situation seriously enough, such clients can make great progress unencumbered by the fear and discouragement that comes with fully developed health challenges.

Coaching for Medical Compliance

As we have discussed before, there is a huge behavioral component to medical compliance. This fact has been recognized by the medical field for quite some time, but what to do about it has been another quandary. One increasingly common approach, especially used by corporations who self-insure, is to seek ways to increase medical compliance. This type of compliance can be measured on limited variables by using blood tests, blood pressure readings, etc. When employee/patients comply, they receive a discount on their share of their health insurance premiums.

To aid in this medical compliance, systems of coaching are gaining popularity. One of the most direct forms of wellness coaching has been systems and services, such as disease management companies, that call patients once a month or so for five or ten minutes, check in with them, and ask if they have been taking their medications and doing their own self-testing/self-treatment properly. This has been a helpful process for some patients. The infrequency of the calls and the severe time limit for questions and/or building an alliance with the coach can, however, handicap this method.

The other aspect of medical compliance is behavioral lifestyle compliance. This is compliance with a lifestyle prescription. In addition to urging compliance with the pharmaceutical prescription and prescribed self-testing/self-treatment directives, there is often a directive to make certain lifestyle improvements—all of which are behavioral. Here, too, the coaches involved in such programs report real benefits to using a coach-approach. They find they are better equipped to establish a trusting relationship, focus the conversation to zero in on key issues (vital with severe time limits), and hold clients accountable in a better way. This is where expanded wellness coaching models and methods step further into the picture. When the coach has more contact time, professional training, and has set up a coaching alliance with their client, a broader range of behavior can be addressed.

We need to look at the effect of having a coaching ally who will address adherence to both treatment programs and the lifestyle prescriptions that accompany them. If over half of what determines our health is our lifestyle, how can we afford not to develop the best systems possible to support people in lasting lifestyle behavioral change?

Coaching On the Comeback Trail

Compassion and empathy with someone who is facing a serious health challenge takes courage. As a wellness coach you have to be willing to feel. You have to be willing to get close enough to your client's experience to realize that it could be you. That with a change in the winds of fate, karma, joss, or whatever you might call it, it could be you. Imagine you are flat on your back in a hospital bed. You have just completed a surgical procedure that felt like a train wreck with you right in the middle of it. Once you become aware enough of what is around you, the first thing you want is contact with other human beings. People often feel lost, sad, and lonely and want connectedness right now! Human contact, human touch—to know that you are not alone means the world to you.

It starts with loved ones who may or may not have been around, or with the kind and caring touch of the hospital staff. Little by little progress is made from that excruciatingly long first walk to the bathroom to sitting in a recliner with oxygen, to cranking up the speed on the treadmill in rehabilitation therapy. Fears are faced continually along the way. There is a yearning for more information about what is normal in the recovery process. Side effects of new medications range from bothersome to terrifying. Fears exaggerate every little physical difficulty.

Not so many years ago cardiac rehabilitation took an approach of rest not exercise. Then the medical field realized that movement was good, even vital to the healing and recovery process. Lifestyle improvement is now seen as an essential component of practically all recovery processes. Journeying out of the land of fear and reclaiming our health, our confidence and our independence is often a long hard walk. Traveling with the support and companionship of others makes the journey easier and helps the person arrive more surely at their successful destination.

Coaching the Re-integration of Work, Family and Self-care

The field of coaching has long specialized in helping people to achieve their goals in their careers and their businesses. Coaches help entrepreneurs to work smarter and more profitably. Coaches help people develop their careers to higher and more satisfying levels. When a person goes through a major health challenge, such as heart surgery, and eventually both needs and wants to return to work, a well-trained wellness coach is in a position to help them do this in a way that is both productive and healthy.

We've all heard stories about remarkable people who, for example, suffered heart attacks and didn't change their lifestyles or way of working one bit. I remember hearing of a high school principal who had an impressive reputation as a hard-charging, high stress, get-things-done-now kind of guy. After his heart attack, at about age 45, he returned to work almost immediately and absolutely reveled in showing everyone how little he had been affected by this blow to his health. He told everyone that the key to success in life was to work hard and when trouble arose, just work harder. He died within a year or two of yet another heart attack. Take a look at the classic movie *All That Jazz!*, for an amazing dramatization of this kind of approach to life.

As part of everyone's rehabilitation process there is a very large behavior change dimension. Compliance with a treatment program means taking medications, doing tests and following up with doctor visits in an effective manner. It also means, in most cases, lots of recommendations for lifestyle change. New diets, new exercise regimens, breathing exercises, relaxation training, using stress management strategies, are all behaviors. In addition to the usual challenge of how to fit these behaviors into a busy life, your client also has to find a way to do more behavioral self-care than ever before. At the same time the client must re-integrate themselves back into the world of work, and to the demands and dynamics of their families. What seemed like a tricky balancing act before may feel like a juggling act in a circus now!

If your client has suddenly been given a shocking message about their health such as we've described here, how they deal with it will depend largely on what stage of readiness for change they are at. It would be easy to assume, as many health care professionals do, that the seriousness of the diagnosis would prompt immediate action yielding all the needed behavioral change. Ah, if it were only true all the time! Astonishingly, some people do not take action.

Your client may have come to you when they are still motivated by their frightful health news. Or they may be at a point where the fire is out, but the health challenge remains. A client's readiness for change and their feelings of grief and loss when looking at their health challenge may all play a complicated role in the individual's motivation to make true changes. A concept that needs to be understood is found in the work of Elizabeth Kubler-Ross (*On Death and Dying*). What we perceive as loss—is loss. The perceived loss of our health activates the same process of grieving that we experience with other losses. The coaching work you do with your client will benefit from integrating what we know about the grieving process with what we know about readiness for change.

R

LIFESTYLE PRESCRIPTION

Dear Health Care Provider:

Your patient is working with a Certified Wellness Coach to improve their life style. Please make your behavior related improvements known to your patient below.

Patients Name: _____   Date: _____

To improve your health I am recommending the following lifestyle behavior improvements:

Restrictions (if any):

I give permission for lifestyle related medical information to be shared with my wellness coach.

_____   _____
      Name of Wellness Coach   Patient Signature

Reproducible Worksheet Masters are available for purchase on CD ROM from Whole Person Associates, 101 W. 2nd St., Suite 203, Duluth, MN 55802, 800-247-6789, www.wholeperson.com.

FIGURE 10.2

Readiness for Change, Grief, and Wellness Coaching

The Five Stages of Grieving and the Loss of Health

1. Denial, Shock and Isolation. The first reaction to learning of illness or death is to deny the reality of the situation. It is a normal reaction to rationalize overwhelming emotions. It is a defense mechanism that buffers the immediate shock. We block out the words and hide from the facts. This is a temporary response that carries us through the first wave of pain. The reality of a health issue has not yet been accepted by the person. He or she feels stunned and bewildered as if everything is "unreal."

2. Anger. As the masking effects of denial and isolation begin to wear, reality and its pain re-emerge. We are not ready. The intense emotion is deflected from our vulnerable core, redirected and expressed instead as anger. The anger may be aimed at inanimate objects, complete strangers, friends or family. Anger may be directed at our loved ones or our God. Rationally, we know they are not to be blamed. Emotionally, however, we may resent God for causing us pain. We feel guilty for being angry, and this makes us more angry. The grief stricken person often lashes out at family, friends, themselves, God, or the world in general. Bereaved people will also experience feelings of guilt or fear during this stage.

3. Bargaining. The normal reaction to feelings of helplessness and vulnerability is often a need to regain control. If only we had sought medical attention sooner. If only we had gotten a second opinion from another doctor. If we changed our diet, maybe we would have gotten well. In this stage, the bereaved asks for a deal or reward from either God, the doctor, or the clergy. Comments like "I'll go to Church every day, if only my health will come back to me" are common.

4. Depression. Depression occurs as a reaction to the changed way of life created by the loss. The bereaved person feels intensely sad, hopeless, drained and helpless. The way we used to view ourselves is missed and thought about constantly. Our reaction relates to the practical implications connected to the change. Sadness and regret predominate. We worry about the cost of treatment and the effect the illness will have on our lives and on those we love. We worry that, in our grief, we have spent less time with others that depend on us. This phase may be eased by simple clarification and reassurance. We may need a bit of helpful cooperation and a few kind words.

5. Acceptance. Acceptance comes when the changes brought upon the person by the loss are stabilized into a new lifestyle. It is not necessarily a mark of bravery to resist the inevitable and to deny ourselves the opportunity to make our peace. This phase is marked by withdrawal and calm. This is not a period of happiness and must be distinguished from depression. Usually, children recover more quickly, while the elderly take the longest. This is a time of integrating new information into a lifestyle or way of being in the world that works for the person.

A Story of Empathy With Loss

While in graduate school an older woman who was a fellow student in the doctoral program told a story about her most profound experience with attempting to empathize with another person. Betty was visiting a dear friend in the hospital who had just had her leg amputated due to her diabetes. Betty was in such pain seeing her friend lying there in misery. She felt the connection with her friend very deeply and searched for something to say. The best she could come forth with was "I know just how you feel."

Her friend's eyes narrowed, anger welled up inside of her and she yelled at Betty "How can you stand there on two good legs and know just how I feel?" Betty felt hit by a cannonball and had regretted her own statement as soon as it had left her mouth. Her heart went down to her feet but then somehow bounced back up, and recovering her sensitivity once again, Betty said, "There is no way I can know what it is like to lose a leg. But I do know what loss, deep loss, is like." Her friend understood Betty's botched initial attempt at empathy, and now felt the true empathy that Betty was showing her. They embraced and cried together.

Betty's story illustrates how we do not have to have the same experience as our client to be able to empathize. How can I be empathic with my morbidly obese client when I've never been overweight in my life? I can do so by drawing upon my common human experience of going through some of the same emotions as my client, but perhaps in a different context. Have I ever been embarrassed, ashamed, or felt like I was being ridiculed by others? Certainly. That becomes the common ground I can draw upon to make empathic statements to my client.

You may find that it is not unusual to be coaching someone whose spouse, or other loved one, is facing a serious health challenge, even a terminal diagnosis. Be a source of support for your client. Help them expand their other sources of support, friends, family and community resources like hospice. Check out the tremendously useful contributions in this area made by Stephen Levine, author of *Who Dies?: An Investigation of Conscious Living and Conscious Dying*. Recommend his book to your clients. Help your client to practice extreme self-care right when they may feel all they can do is give to their loved one. If they empty their own reserves of health they will have even less available to help their loved one.

Prevention takes on a new dimension once a health challenge arises. Instead of exercising to feel better and to prevent the onset of some health challenge in the future, self-care behaviors need to be done now, or there may be much more immediate losses. Lung capacity may not return unless certain breathing exercises are done regularly. Muscle atrophy may increase, joint flexibility may be lost, stamina may not return if the prescribed movement program is not maintained. Blood sugar levels need to be stabilized through consistent and proper diet and exercise or insulin levels will shift the person into immediate and negative consequences.

Perhaps a more insidious situation occurs when your client can return to their old lifestyle patterns and seem to get away with it for a while. There are no immediately apparent consequences, so there is a natural tendency to return to business (and life) as usual. Even though your client may have been told that they will pay later for not changing their lifestyle behavior, the old habits are most likely to return.

Work/life balance takes on new and even deeper meaning when your client is recovering from surgery and/or dealing with a new and major health challenge. Very often a major contributor to the health challenge they face is the former strategy of sacrificing one's health for one's job, or for the benefit of others and not taking enough care of themselves. A pattern of letting self-care go in order to have more time for work, family, and community may have become deeply ingrained and socially reinforced. Now the sudden realization that self-care behaviors are more critical than ever may or may not produce the needed change.

Every client will have a unique experience when it comes time to begin re-integrating themselves back into their world of work. Self-employed people make up a larger portion of the population than ever before. When they don't work, there is, of course, little income. The same may be true for many blue-collar workers as well. Not everyone has disability insurance, qualifies for worker's compensation, or has solid company or union benefits behind them. In addition to the obvious pressure to restore income, there are a variety of both external and internal pressures.

Pressures to Return to Work and Resume Previous Ways	
External Pressures	**Internal Pressures**
• Restore Income—both realistically and pressure from family to do so • Return to former style of work-priority over self-care priority • Resume former pace of work and catch up on projects • Resume former levels of performance	• Regain self-respect and perceived respect of others • "Prove" to self that "it's not that bad" • Reassure self that all is not lost (abilities, etc.) • Identifying heavily with work as defining self and self-worth • Fend off fear of death by regaining a sense of control

TABLE 10.1

Coaching Your Client to Respond to Internal and External Pressures

As you can see in Table 10.1, the internal pressures affecting your client's return to work are not all intrinsically negative. Restoring income and self-respect are certainly wonderful things. The more negative internal forces are largely found around fear and sense of self. This is why we have emphasized more work on internal wellness. There is real value in the exploration of the self, and the deeper work on self that we have referred to here.

Be sensitive to the possibility that your clients will push themselves too hard and too fast to return to work and resume previous workloads and performance standards. Look for signs of desperation and an excessive sense of urgency. Help them gain some insights and self-understanding. Ask them powerful questions to challenge their perceptions of deadlines and expectations, which they may be attributing to outside sources, but are really within themselves.

There are times when there is a great deal of external pressure and not all of it may be healthy, or at least not in the best interests of your client's health. There are certainly workplaces that care very much about employees and value them, just as there are those that do not. Pressures can come from supervisors and from co-workers.

Some of your most valuable wellness coaching may really be about assertiveness. Help your client to be in touch with their own self-worth, to value their own health and well-being as a true priority. To protect this they may have to forge new boundaries that were not in place before. Your client may have to re-train other people in how to treat them. The do anything for others person may have to quit putting their own needs last and develop the fine art of saying no more often. Coach your client through this process. Help them experiment with new behavior in this area and help them process their experience as they attempt to put it in place.

Coach your client through the emotions of dealing with new physical limitations — and dealing realistically with them. They may simply not have the strength or endurance they had before. They may have to tread in what is for them new territory, and ask for help more often. Help them develop the essential skill of strategic delegation and coach them through the experience of implementing that skill. As always, be their ally as they explore what is now a new way of being in the world.

Health Challenge Specialization

In your healthcare work, or as a special niche in the wellness coaching you choose to do, you may be working with people with particular health challenges. In the United States the statistics on the occurrence of obesity, cancer, heart disease and diabetes (with it's epidemic numbers) are an indication of the tremendous need.

You may or may not have personal experience with one of these challenges yourself. Frequently the wellness coaching classes and trainings I have led have included coaches and healthcare workers whose interest in health and wellness was initiated by their own personal experience. We discovered years ago in the addictions field, you don't have to be a recovered drug addict or alcoholic to be an effective counselor to someone with that current challenge. Having experience in the area does help though, to establish trust, inspire hope, set intrinsic empathy, and familiarize the coach with the life of a person with that health challenge.

As a wellness coach with or without first-hand experience with a particular health challenge, you need to familiarize yourself with what your clients have as their personal and medical experience. When coaching a post-heart surgery client, you might benefit greatly from knowing what someone goes through with blood thinning medications. Find out what their medication is, what the generic name for it is, how it works, how blood levels are tested, what that testing is called, what scores they have been told to shoot for, what the most common side effects are, etc. That may sound like a lot of detail, but, for example, when your client begins talking with you about how they are working with a nutritionist to eat healthy, yet reduce their vitamin K (which increases the clotting factor in the blood) it would be good if you knew what they were talking about! Your specialized knowledge is not there for you to make any treatment decisions (unless that is your qualified healthcare job). It is there to provide empathy and understanding and increase trust. I'm more likely to trust a coach who understands my cholesterol score, or blood sugar level numbers in light of my treatment goals than one to whom I have to explain something so basic.

Let the Other Pros Help Too

The approach to coaching in this book and the Wellness Mapping 360°™ approach are based on the concept that much of what you do with any person with a health challenge will follow the same effective methods of good coaching. Support your client and the (other) healthcare professionals in what they do, and be a great coach!

Your client most likely has available to them a whole host of professional services that can help them with their health challenge, major surgery rehabilitation and even their return to work. Rehabilitation therapists, occupational therapists, job counselors, and social workers are among those who may be available for your client's needs. Your client may need assistance navigating the system to find the help they need. If you are specializing in coaching people with health challenges, become very familiar with the professional options available in your community, or, if you are coaching remotely, coach your client through the process of discovering for themselves what assets are available. Again, be their coaching ally and refer often to other professionals who can help your client.

Wellness Mapping 360°™ in Health Coaching – A Case Example

A part of the *Mindset Shift* is to understand that you are stepping out of the expert role and into the support or ally role. You are always coaching your client toward understanding or developing what they need. You support the client to find the information and resources they need. You help the client develop their personal visions and create the map that will guide them there. The Wellness Mapping 360°™ model gives both the coach and the client the environment for this to occur.

Here is an example of what a completed Wellness Map might look like for a client who is facing a health challenge. In this example we will talk about the experience of a man in his mid-fifties who has undergone successful heart surgery for mitral valve repair. This fictitious case is based partly on my own experience, and also, in part, upon the experience of others I have known.

Client Description: 56 year old male whom we will call Ken Black. He is remarried, with children and stepchildren who are grown and on their own, but remain nearby the small town he lives in. His wife is very supportive and understanding. Ken is a college biology professor who successfully underwent mitral valve repair surgery five months ago. This open-heart procedure was preceded by an experience with congestive heart failure where his lungs were filling with fluid, threatening his life. Ken was in very good health before the surgery and exercised regularly and enjoyed hiking and many outdoor activities.

Thirty-six sessions of cardiac rehabilitation (CR) were very beneficial for Ken. He completed this program recently and has been having a hard time maintaining the progress and regularity he achieved physically while attending the CR session three times a week. Ken is also finding that returning to work is not as easy as he thought it would be. The new school year brought its usual stress and accelerated pace for which he was not ready.

Ken is looking to your coaching help adjust to his full-time work, and to balance it with an adequate program of healthy self-care that will aid with his recovery.

My Wellness Map—Life Vision and Focus Tool
KEN BLACK

1. Life Vision—Either on your own or working with your coach, ar-

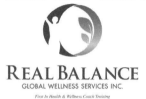

rive at a statement that sums up your idea of what it would look like to be living your life to the fullest and functioning at your best. Be realistic and yet, inspiring!

My Life's Wellness Vision:

I want to regain my health and vital-ity so I can return to the active outdoor lifestyle I love and continue to be there for the ones I love. I see myself as an older man who is still able to hike, camp, swim, fish, and even do wilderness canoe trips when I'm old enough to take my (future) grandchildren along with me!

2. Current Life Status—Summarize what your current life is like. Do not be discouraged or judgmental with yourself—just be honest.

> *I've got to say that despite all I've been through this year, that life is pretty good. I enjoy wonderful support from my wife and children, and from friends as well. I've been recovering well, but still am working at regaining my former strength and endurance. I still get winded going uphill, more than before. I still fret over any little thing that goes wrong, like feeling light-headed, gaining weight suddenly, etc. I'm still fifteen pounds heavier than before I went in for surgery.*

Returning to work has been tough. The small college I work at is under-funded and in our department the chairwoman seems to be more worried about how many students we at-tract and retain than about delivering a quality education. I wanted a reduced number of classes to teach but didn't get it. There seems to be little accommodation for my health by my chair, and my colleagues. The students are great, but there's just too many of them! And now I have to do all this exercising, taking time to rest and so forth. I feel like I don't have time for all of it.

Take a deep breath, relax and ask yourself "What would have to change for me to achieve my life vision?"

> I need to get some consistency. I'm afraid of losing ground already on what I achieved in rehab. I want to get my lungs back! I think that I've got to find a way to handle work better, not stress over it so much, and take care of myself better.

3. Areas of Focus — To make my life vision a reality I choose to focus on the following areas of my life. For maximum success, prioritize no more than five areas and make those areas the ones you are most ready to address. Suggested lifestyle improvements from healthcare providers and results from wellness assessments or health risk assessments can also be listed. You might want to work together with your coach to determine these areas.

1. Balancing work demands and self-care activities

2. Exercising

3. Managing stress

4. Following through on all medical appointments and taking meds on schedule

Areas of Focus Sheet

Area of Focus One — To make my vision real I want to focus on the

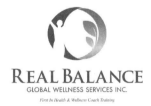

following area. Choose an area from #3 of the Life Vision and Focus Page that you are most ready to work on or because you feel you need it the most, or because it is easy and you just want to get the ball rolling.

Focus area: Balancing work demands and self-care activities

A. Desires: What do you want or how would you like it to be? Write in your own words, "What are your stated desires for this area of focus in your life?"

This is good to state as both an immediate action your want to see happen (for example, I want to lose ten pounds) and in a longer-term, more motivational action (for example, I want to be able to go on a very physically active vacation this summer).

I want to schedule my day and week with self-care a priority over work.

I want to meet my work obligations while taking excellent care of myself.

B. Current Location: Where do you see yourself currently in this area of your life?

Right now this is where I'm at regarding this area of focus: (List whatever describes your present situation. For example you could list your current percent body fat; number of hours of sleep/night; 1-10 scale self-ratings of situations or levels of conditioning, etc.)

Currently I am exercising too little and not getting enough rest to improve my physical condition. I have gained five pounds since ending cardiac rehab classes and am not increasing my stamina. I am feeling very stressed by a demanding workload. My requests for some consideration of my recovery are not being responded to. I feel very unsupported at work and under pressure.

C. The Path: What do you need to do? What do you need to do or what needs to change in your life for you to realize your desire for this area in your life?

Describe what needs to change in this area of your life for you to attain your desires. State the changes needed as specifically as you can.

1. I need to make my health and self-care my #1 priority. I need to believe that myself and hold it in mind first every day.

2. I need to increase the amount of self-care activities that I do, and be very consistent.

3. I need to get more understanding and support from my department for my health recovery.

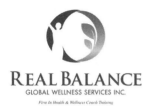

Areas of Focus Sheet
Page Two

REAL BALANCE
GLOBAL WELLNESS SERVICES INC.
First In Health & Wellness Coach Training

D. Committed Course: What are you making a commitment to do? Work with your coach to create realistic and attainable action steps that will move you towards the desired outcome for your chosen life area. Choose an initial step to make that will get you moving. Like a map, chart your course to your chosen change. Once again being specific is important. Write down what you will do, when it will be completed by, and how you will communicate the accomplishment to your coach. Work with your coach to arrive at strategies that are challenging enough without being too much.

What You Will Do	Duration	When	Check in Method
Step 1. I will write down my planned self-care activities (exercise, rest, etc.) and what I actually did.	For one month and then review with my coach	Each AM and each PM	I will e-mail my coach each Monday and Friday and will also discuss this during my coaching appointments
Step 2. I will keep a wellness journal. There I will write down what I am experiencing with seeking balance between work and increased self-care.	For one month and then review with my coach	Five days a week	I will report in on how the journaling is going and any insights I gain during my weekly coaching session
Step 3. I will gather my courage and have a very honest conversation with my chairperson about my recovery and my need to prioritize my health	Once, or more times if needed	As soon as the schedule of my chairperson permits	I will e-mail my coach within one week and report on scheduling progress. I will prepare for the meeting in my coaching appt. and report on the meeting in my next coaching appt.

TABLE 10.3

Brainstorm here:

Be assertive about getting on Chair's schedule. Push for talking with her within one week. Don't let it wait. Keep a wellness journal on my personal computer, include pictures, etc. to make it more fun and positive.

E. Challenges: What are you up against? List what obstacles are in your way or what you believe could prevent you from reaching your desired destination.

High stress environment in my department. With the new school year starting there has been little accommodation for my recovery in terms of work load, and there has been resentment expressed by both chairperson and colleagues regarding the time I take to exercise and rest.

On my side, I don't like to feel like I am not pulling my weight, my fair share of the work when we are all under pressure. I want to help my department face its larger challenges of lack of funding, etc. At times I fear losing my job when that realistically is not likely to happen.

Go back and forth from periods of too much self-care neglect (where I end of feeling fatigued, and make little recovery progress), to periods of inadequate attention to my work.

F. Strategies To Meet The Challenges: Ways to overcome the hurdles. With your coach develop strategies that you can use to make adjustments in your life to overcome or get around things that hold you back from your committed course of action. (For example: when under a work deadline I will make my exercise session briefer, but not skip it.)

1. Increasing communication with my chair and others in the department. Most of them know little if anything about valve surgery and expect me to recuperate just as fast as someone they know who had by-pass surgery, which is significantly different. Have more formal and informal conversations with all in my department.

2. Ask for the support I need. Tell others what I need and very specifically how they can be of help.

3. Using my calendar more to plan ahead of time for my self-care activities instead of just fitting them in where I can, when I think of it. Journaling about the work/life balance and keeping track of it. Keeping work/life/recovery balance a central area of focus for my coaching.

G. Sources of Support: Who can share this journey with you or support your journey? State specifically who or what your sources of support, encouragement, and accountability are as you follow this area of focus on your wellness map into new territory.

1. Talk more with my wife about all of this. She can handle it, and is very supportive. She is also a great source of ideas.

2. One colleague, Bill, has been through some serious health challenges of his own, including the onset of diabetes. He seems to exercise quite religiously. I will reach out to him too.

3. My friends outside of the university department are very positive. I will avoid complaining to them about my struggles for support in the department and will do more to enjoy our friendships.

This same process would then be completed with each area of focus that Ken indicated (exercise, managing stress, following through on all medical appointments and taking meds on schedule).

The coach would then meet at the designated times with Ken and review his progress and explore what gets in the way. Once the Wellness Map is set up it is easy to see when the client accomplishes what they set out to do and this is a time to celebrate.

> *We are what we think. All that we are arises with our thoughts. With our thoughts, we make the world.*

> **—Siddhartha Gautama**, *The Buddha*

Chapter 11

Wellness Coaching In Action

Today, almost 95 percent of the things we spend our money on—which most of us think of as necessities—were not seen around when many of us were born: television sets, airline travel, Disneyland vacations, high-fashion clothing, stereos, DVDs, air conditioners, personal computers, day care, movies, fast-food restaurants, dry cleaning, Internet access, to name a few. The same will happen with wellness.

—Paul Zane Pilzer
The Wellness Revolution, p. 47

Wellness Coaching: Destination Unknown—Possibilities Endless

Closely observing and actively participating in the wellness field since 1979 has been a joy. Watching it go through it's own metamorphosis has been at once interesting, puzzling, astonishing, and continually surprising. I've seen it labeled a dream, a temporary trend, a wave, and even a tidal wave. It's been called essential, superfluous, vital, unnecessary, flakey, evidence-based, touchy-feely, and the only way we're ever going to make an impact on healthcare costs. I've spoken around the world on wellness and found that it is here to stay.

Wellness programming works! The effectiveness of wellness programs in reducing health risks and affecting the bottom line are now substantially documented. An exhaustive review of the evidence appears in Larry Chapman's book Proof Positive: The Practitioner's Guide To ROI and Program Development, published by The Wellness Councils of America (WELCOA). Chapman sees wellness programs as being capable of both quick and long-term positive returns on investment. As more coaching components are added to wellness programs gathering data on their effectiveness is essential.

The visibility of wellness coaching seems to be increasing rapidly in recent times. The services that are being called wellness coaching come in many shapes and sizes. Just as in the coaching field when managers became coaches and merely did what they always did and just changed their title, some wellness professionals take on the new title of coach and continue to do individual work as best they can. Others pursue coach training vigorously and find great benefit in it. The upside is that people in corporate wellness programs, many medical fields, insurance companies and individuals as well, see the value of wellness coaching. It's almost like there are many chefs out there who are having tremendous creative fun combining the two ingredients of wellness and coaching in ways never thought of before!

The trend toward the individualization of wellness is clear. As more wellness professionals bring more one-on-one focus into their work they are turning consulting and educating into coaching. Also, coaches with an interest in the health and wellness fields are discovering ways to apply their coach training to the wellness arena. A thorough overview of this ever-changing field is like describing a sunset or perhaps a sunrise that is constantly changing before your eyes.

Since the publication of our first edition of this book (2007) we have seen wellness and health coaching go from a young profession to what is now considered a "best practice" in any wellness program. (Edington, 2013) Wellness coaching is seen as the delivery mechanism for the individual services of such programs. Optum Health has been tracking the prevalence of wellness coaching used by organizations since 2007. It rose in use from 44% to 56% by 2009. In their 2011 survey they state that they found eight out of ten organizations offering wellness coaching. Wellness coaching is now an integral part of the health promotion landscape in the United States.

Corporate Applications

The powerful return on investment (ROI) for comprehensive wellness programs has convinced the vast majority of larger organizations to invest in wellness. (Chapman, 2013) Now as we saw in the Optum Health report, almost 80% of the time wellness coaching is part of the program. Many organizations still use the telephonic coaching services offered by their large health insurance carrier, but others are having their wellness program staff (health educators, nurses, fitness trainers, etc.) trained as wellness coaches. Wellness coaching companies such as Wellness Coaches USA actually insert a wellness coach right into a contracted worksite so that they can build connections with employees and make wellness coaching maximally accessible.

More and more of the large disease management companies have moved beyond a focus on medical compliance/adherence and are infusing their coaching services with well-thought-out behavioral change methods. Large and even smaller health insurance companies are offering wellness coaching to their members to help hold down healthcare costs. For self-insuring organizations holding down those costs from year to year is imperative. Including wellness coaching as a vital part of their wellness programs is an effective strategy. As the healthcare landscape changes and becomes more competitive offering wellness coaching as a benefit makes one company more attractive over another.

Responding to the pressure to hold down healthcare costs and improve employee health the wellness educators, nurses, and others who are often leading these wellness programs are increasingly being directed to deliver wellness coaching services. As a result they seek quality wellness coach training to plug their own educational gap in behavioral change skills.

Employee Assistant Programs (EAP's) are increasingly offering wellness coaching services as one of their products. EAP counselors often include people with masters degrees in counseling and psychology, or registered dieticians, nurses, and health educators, giving them excellent backgrounds to develop into effective wellness coaches.

Coaching in corporations and large organizations has been well established for about twenty years now. Whether it is called leadership coaching, business coaching, executive coaching or simply life coaching, these organizations have found real value in having coaches available to their personnel. While many of these coaches have often worked on "work-life balance" issues with their clients, there has been an increasing recognition of the need for coaches well-trained in wellness coaching to be added to the list of coaching services available. The physical as well as the mental/emotional health of managers and executives is critical to organizational effectiveness and productivity.

The ideal organization focuses on developing a culture of wellness that reaches from the top to the bottom. Comprehensive wellness programs include opportunities, facilities, and services for education, healthy-living skill development (like cooking skills for busy people), and wellness coaching to deliver the individualization of wellness. Buy-in at the top sets in motion policies and systems that allow wellness to thrive. When managers see the value in having their employees who report to them experiencing better health they are more supportive of the participation of these employees in wellness programming and coaching. When these managers experience the benefits of these same wellness services they thrive and offer even more support.

The Question of Incentives

Some organizations attempt to incentivize participation in wellness programs through offering discounts on the employee's health insurance premiums. This controversial practice opens the door for some employees to see a wellness coach, and for others it creates a reaction where the employee participates to comply with the requirement (to get the discount). In this case the employee sometimes resents being there and presents a real challenge for the wellness coach to create a positive coaching alliance with them.

This practice is currently wide-spread and the challenge is for organizations to present the wellness coach as ally not enemy. For the coach the challenge is to honor their client's frustration, empathize with their point of view and offer the opportunity to make maximal advantage of the services they are there to experience anyway.

The effectiveness of such incentives is under great scrutiny and is the focus of a huge debate in the health promotion industry. Those who argue the case for intrinsic motivation (See Daniel Pink's book Drive: The Surprising Truth About What Motivates Us) would say that most people "learn how to play the game" and then quit once they've gotten their prize (discount).

Applications In Medical Settings

The emerging field of Lifestyle Medicine has assembled more than ample evidence that one's lifestyle behavior affects the course of an illness. (see www.lifestylemedicine.org) Wellness is not just about prevention, it is about helping people experience their health challenges (chronic illness, surgery recovery, etc.) with the highest levels of wellness possible for them. Lifestyle Medicine is showing us how behavioral health is. From better medical compliance helping a person with diabetes to thrive, to the heart patient who's coaching post-cardiac rehabilitation helps them be able to continue to exercise regularly and improve their diet. Wellness coaching is helping people with smoking cessation, weight loss, the better management of stress, and so much more. People with health challenges often make up the majority of clients for wellness coaches (and what we call health coaches) are working with.

Medical practices, hospitals and other medical settings are starting to see the value of integrating wellness coaches into their efforts at improving quality of care. As the medical world is nudged forward by new forces such as payment based on improved performance outcomes, shared decision making, patient-centered care, and more, wellness coaches have a new role to play as part of the team. Physical therapy practices are seeing the value of the wellness coach approach in helping their patients be more engaged with the home exercises they prescribe. Dieticians are finding coaching to be the key to helping their clients succeed at implementing the new eating programs that they recommend. It is all evolving, but extremely exciting times for wellness coaches in the world of medicine and allied health.

Expanding the HRA paradigm

In Chapter Seven we spoke at length about health risk appraisals and the various ways they are used to help people take charge of their own wellness. Certainly one of the most common wellness programming scenarios is when an HRA instrument is applied widely to an employee population and the results are shared in some form of feedback process. In this setting wellness coaching can be put into action allowing the employee with a health risk to work in multiple sessions with a well-trained wellness coach. Here are some suggestions to consider for making HRAs and wellness coaching a positive piece of the company's wellness program:

- Hire companies with well-trained wellness/health coaches who process HRA results with employees either in-person, or on the telephone.

- Another option is to train your in-house staff who work with HRA's in wellness coaching.

- Give employees more than one session. Multiple sessions allow true coaching to take place with opportunity for change, accountability, and the value of the coaching alliance.

- Make coaching sessions as long and as often as feasible.

- Take "Readiness for Change" into consideration as you develop your program.

- Make wellness coaching available to all, not just high-risk employees.

Wellness coaches may work with especially valuable employees to help prevent burnout and retain them as healthy employees longer. They may be assigned to work with employees identified as being at high-risk medically in an attempt to curtail the usage of a high percentage of healthcare costs by high-risk individuals. Or they may take the approach that it is less expensive to keep healthy employees healthy by the preventative power of living healthier wellness lifestyles.

As an in-house wellness coach you may have the opportunity to work face-to-face more often with your clients. This model works well for large companies who are centrally located. For companies with sites in many geographic locations telephone-based coaching is a good alternative. This can be achieved either through on-staff coaches or through contracting with independent coaches or coaching services.

Organizations may also find that it may be more cost-effective for them to outsource wellness coaching services rather than have the added expenses of full-time employees and providing them benefits packages, etc. If the teleconference style of coaching is likely to be the norm the coaches can be anywhere and still connect with the employee who needs coaching.

Taking It Directly to the Consumer

Eleven years ago Paul Pilzer wrote about the emerging *Wellness Revolution*, boldly predicting it would be the next trillion dollar industry. In 2007 he updated his work with a second edition where he estimated that what he very inclusively called wellness had already grown from a 200 billion dollar industry to a 500 billion dollar money maker. It would be easy to guess that Pilzer's prediction of a trillion dollar industry has come true. Much of it comes down to the demand of a population that is both aging and extremely health conscious.

Demographics rule much of the wellness field. When we look at the epidemiological factors of illness and the sociological factors influencing behavioral change we see that who, what and where are big questions to answer. In the United States the sheer numbers of the baby boom generation are astounding. We must remember that World War Two did not have this same effect everywhere else in the world. Much of Europe experienced great loss of life while we were booming. The bulge in the population that the boomers push up in the U.S. is absent in these countries.

The baby-boom generation continues to have an enormous impact on healthcare in America and is putting tremendous stress on the medical system. In addition to remedial care demands, the desire for more and more health and wellness-related products is skyrocketing. "The economic impact of the baby boomers on wellness is even stronger than their numbers suggest—because this group is behaving differently than any prior generation. Boomers are refusing to passively accept the aging process." (Pilzer, The Wellness Revolution, p. 42)

Among the customers in the fitness center, alongside the trim younger bodies are women with long grey hair down over their shoulders and men whose hair, what they have left of it, is also turning more and more silver. You see it everywhere. Boomers on the bike paths, out dancing, filling the Yoga classes, and snatching up all the copies of health, fitness, and spa magazines. Vitamins fly off the shelf, while demand for organic and natural foods continues to amaze us all. And, the demand is coming not only from the aging baby-boom generation, but from younger minds who see the value in living a wellness lifestyle, being active and are more at ease about self-pampering in spas, etc.

Elsewhere in the world there is also tremendous interest in wellness. As we see in the U.S., there are overlaps between alternative medicine (a.k.a. complimentary medicine, integrative medicine), holistic health, and wellness. From spas in Thailand and Brazil to wellness resource websites in Poland, we see expanding application of new ideas in wellness and more and more interest in the self-employed coach.

In-house and Outsourced Wellness Coaches

Many coaches are self-employed. By either applying previously gained knowledge from the world of business, or by rapidly learning the ropes of entrepreneurship, coaches can bring many good ideas to the wellness industry. The question is: how can you position your services to attract people interested in wellness.

About a quarter of the thousands of wellness coaches we have trained are self-employed. Many of them are attracted to the independence of such work. Many are attracted to holistic health, fitness, and the positive nature of the wellness field. Some have made their own remarkable journey from illness to health and attribute a great share of their health to their success at lifestyle improvement.

Entrepreneurial coaches face the challenge of continuously having to educate their potential customers on what wellness coaching is and how it can benefit them. Their toughest challenge is finding individuals who are willing to pay for these services out of their own pocket. A common strategy is to complement your strictly independent work with alliances formed with referral organizations. Wellness coaches plug their services into wellness programs already offering services to employees. By being one of these out-sourced coaches a more steady base of clients can be found. Wellness coaches are becoming valued by medical practices and as reimbursement strategies and policies evolve this will become easier and easier.

Many coaches find that their clients connect with them because they have seen them speak or present somewhere. There has been some kind of personal exposure that is far more powerful and more trust building than any printed or electronic marketing can create.

One way to attract the wellness consumer directly is by creating attractive wellness-oriented retreats, workshops or *play-shops*. Make the experience fun, practical, relaxing, and even pampering. Teach people extreme self-care by allowing them to experience some of it. Experiment with the format and find what works for you and your clientele. Half-day, whole day, or weekend resort "get-away" types of retreats may work for your focus clientele. Create the experience around attractive themes and ones the consumer can relate to. Perhaps partner with a colleague or with a professional event planner and do it right! The workshop itself is providing a great service. If people find they can connect with you and are attracted to you as a coach new clients will result. Think of reaching out with your services beyond your local area. It's a big world out there!

Some Self-Employed Wellness Coaching Business Tips

- Grow your coaching business (not "practice") as you can. Consider starting part-time while you gain traction.

- Call it what it is. Name your business something that people understand right way. Avoid the temptation to go with your favorite, but esoteric, name.

- Say it clear, say it now. Be able to articulate with laser-like ability exactly what services you offer, how people benefit from them and what sets you apart.

- Keep the door open. Answering machine messages should clearly state your own name, the name of your business, and be a combination of professional, warm, and inviting. Put your business phone number on the home page of your website where potential clients can find it effortlessly. Don't come across like you are more concerned with your own privacy than you are about being of service.

- Diversify. You are not just a coach. You are bringing all that YOU are to the world. What other skills and talents do you have to offer? Training, consultation, speaking, etc., bring in much needed income and also drive clients to your coaching services. Offer products to the public in ways that do not conflict ethically with your work with clients.

- Learn the business of business. You can do a lot on your own, but also consider courses in coaching attraction/marketing offered by professional coaching schools, and services of private marketing experts and teachers (for example: www. helpingthehelper.com).

- Do what you are best at. Determine when it just isn't worth it for you to do it yourself. Instead of sitting at home learning how to build websites and program HTML, get out and promote yourself in public. Hire others to handle time consuming tasks or ones where someone else's expertise would give you better results.

- Create your own team. Hire a mentor coach. Have great business resources available such as a good webmaster, accountant, a reliable place for your printing, etc. Have great resources available for your own self-care (now needed more than ever): massage therapist, holistic healthcare providers, fitness facilities/resources, spa access, etc.

- Co-create mutual alliances. Develop a network of helping professionals that you refer your clients to (fitness trainers, nutritionists, physicians, psychotherapists, career counselors, acupuncturists, etc.), and develop relationships with them where they are referring to you as well. Don't do business with people who don't want to do business!

- Remember that you are not your work. You are not your cash flow! You own the business, don't let it own you. Avoid over-identifying with your business. Focus and work smart, but have a life—preferably one with fun, grace, and adventure! It all makes you more attractive as a coach anyway.

- Custom fit to your clientele. Consider new and different ways to size, shape, package and custom-fit your services to the people you serve. Experiment with modifying the old standard times and dates for appointment times.

- Coach clients with health challenges. Most wellness coaches find that about 70-80% of their clients already have some sort of chronic illness or condition. By coaching people to thrive with diabetes, heart disease, hypertension, hyperlipidemia, and many other conditions you reach a huge market and make your services available to people who really need them. Again, wellness is not just about prevention anymore!

The Wellness Revolution Rolls On

As lifestyle medicine research has continued to show us the importance of our lifestyle on our health and well-being, the demand for wellness products and services has continued to grow. "Until now, most people were told to accept their wellness deficiencies as part of the aging process, as though there were nothing they could do about them." (Pilzer, p. 57) Now people are quicker to question this assumption and to seek out ways to live their lives with more health and vitality.

Our wellness coaching challenge is not that of "marketing," but of "market development." We market products and services people are already familiar with. We have to do market development to educate consumers as to what our products and services are and how they can benefit them. We are poised to ride an immense economic wave, but the public has to be aware of what we have to offer them.

Positioning wellness coaching is the challenge we all share.

- Position wellness coaching as the resource for lasting lifestyle improvement.

- Position wellness coaching as an ally to the healthcare professionals who want to see their patients thrive.

- Include wellness coaching as part of lifestyle medicine, helping people affect the course of their health challenge through lifestyle improvement.

- Demonstrate that wellness coaching has the kinds of results that show that taking wellness one-on-one is highly effective.

- Provide quality services, collect sound statistics, and get the message out to those who need to know.

New Venues!

Get creative with your wellness coaching marketing development. Go where no coach has gone before! Look for potential places to attract clients or cultivate referrals. Through alliances the wellness coach becomes part of a team. Consider these new venues for wellness coaching:

- Fitness facilities. Workout clubs of all kinds abound. Some of them may be open to having you do a free talk for their members. You may be able to connect with fitness trainers there for mutual referrals. You may even be able to sell the idea of wellness coaching as a service that can be effortlessly added by the facility.

- Health stores. Natural foods stores are growing in superstore proportion. Many have public education programs and even training/presentation rooms available.

- Public athletic clubs. Outdoors clubs.

- Senior citizen centers where public programs happen all the time. Many active seniors are great business/medical contacts.

- Spas and day-spas. The huge public interest in "all things spa" can be capitalized on. Many spas are limited in their services and see themselves primarily as hospitality (hotel) businesses. It is worth exploring how open they are to wellness services for their clients. When they do buy in, they are inexpensively adding your out-sourced service to their clients for very little, if any, expense to themselves. Many of the internationally famous "big name" spas already have full time staff who do wellness coaching. While getting hired there is a long shot, many hundreds of other spas are worth checking out and having conversations with.

Finding the Niche Within the Niche

No matter how you pronounce it, niche marketing can be highly effective. While "wellness" coaching might be considered a niche, how can you set yourself apart even within this very broad area of lifestyle improvement? The challenge here is to be focused without eliminating too many potential clients. Who is your market? Your market may not just be people you are absolutely comfortable with, identify with, or can relate to. While all of that is nice to have in a client, can you really afford to be that restrictive? Perhaps a little stretching and growing would be a good thing for you as a coach, and as a person. Ask yourself, "What holds me back from coaching this variety of client?

It's fine to go with the strength of your own experience, just be vigilant at keeping your story and your client's separate. Your "story" in life can be an advantage. My fifty-five year old friend who coaches people about "retiring well," both personally and financially, will probably get more trusting clients than a twenty-five year old trying to reach the same market. Many of the coaches I've trained have been attracted to wellness coaching from their own experiences with their own health challenges. Cancer survivors, coaches who are diabetic, who have been through heart surgery, who have been successful with weight loss issues, etc., can carry those experiences into developing a coaching niche where knowledge and empathy are very high.

Choose your niche based upon a combination of it really and truly being something you are passionate about and one where there really is a market for it. Does society value what you have to offer? Ask are there ways I can reach a sufficient number of people to serve who need what I offer in this niche? In short, is the niche big enough? What we know for sure is that wellness coaching is becoming an important part of our world as people and businesses strive to become healthier and to reduce the cost of health care.

A non-doer is very often a critic-that is, someone who sits back and watches doers, and then waxes philosophically about how the doers are doing. It's easy to be a critic, but being a doer requires effort, risk, and change.

—Wayne Dyer

271

Afterword: Quantum Soup

This is truly a new batch of soup we are creating in the merger of wellness and coaching. Lasting lifestyle behavioral change is the taste we are trying to attain. No one is sure of the recipe, except that it should have lots of mindset shift, quite a few cups of coaching competencies and a broth that is rich in wellness foundational principles. This is a soup that will come out of every kitchen a bit different, with flavors from bland to spicy. Predicting all the variations would be like trying to predict the future. It is very exciting to anticipate all that will be created. My hope is that it will all be very nourishing.

In *The New Physics for the Twenty-First Century*, edited by Gordon Fraser, it is said that the Universe was a tiny bowl of Quantum Soup until a fraction of a second after the Big Bang. Well, it may be a bit pretentious to compare our fledgling wellness field with the creation of the universe, but have fun and think about it. The desire for greater levels of health in the world is met with the staggering illness statistics we see despite incredible efforts to make a difference. Two forces in separate orbits, like the medical world and the behavioral world, finally intersect like never before, and BANG! We can only hope the new creation will serve us all well.

Behavioral medicine has been around for a long time. As a psychologist I felt very gratified by the progress I saw in clients that I helped with stress-related disorders. Biofeedback, relaxation training, psychotherapy and other approaches all helped. In hospitals psychologists and other behavioral experts continue to make enormous and valuable contributions. What wellness coaching is doing is making the competencies of behavioral change available to more people who are in a variety of helping capacities. We have found ways to extract essential elements of behavioral change, that, combined with a growth-oriented way of practicing yields lifestyle changing results.

It reminds me of days long ago in graduate school when I saw how Robert Carkhuff and Bernard Berenson *(Beyond Counseling and Therapy)* expanded the work of Carl Rogers. They identified three necessary and sufficient conditions that are related to a positive outcome in therapy: acceptance of the client, accurate empathy and congruence on the therapist's part. Perhaps we are evolving a set of competencies through coaching that can serve us the same way in the wellness field.

You are presented with a world of tremendous opportunity. Those feeling the drudgery of illness care are being reinvigorated by both a growth-oriented way of doing healthcare, and a growth-oriented way of living. There will always be a need for remedial care, to say the very least. It is just so exciting to see us going further "upstream" into the land of prevention. It is an inside-out job. As you work on your own personal growth, mind, body, spirit and the connectedness to your environment, you become a person who can help others to grow as well.

Second Edition Soup

Well into the second decade of the new millennium it's hard for me to describe the sense of gratification I feel when observing how wellness coaching has grown. When we look over our shoulders at the thousands of wellness coaches we've trained around the world through Real Balance Global Wellness Services, Inc. and The Wellness Coach Training Institute (www.realbalance.com) and see the difference they are making in people's lives there is amazement, awe and gratitude.

Through the case studies our students write as part of their certification process we've seen client's lives not just improved, but literally saved. I think of a middle-aged male client whose dietician/coach worked with him to finally improve his eating behavior after fourteen years of struggling with diabetes. He managed to pull himself back from the brink of renal failure, going from maxing out his insulin pump every day to a high level of successful management that thrilled his physician. Time and time again we have seen how people benefit from having a relationship with a true wellness ally.

Now we see wellness coaching being recognized as an essential component of comprehensive wellness programs. We've come a long, long way since the first wellness coaching presentations I gave at The National Wellness Conference in the late 1990's.

Our work today is to not just train more coaches, but to provide support for all the wellness coaches out there. We will continue to develop new tools and improved methodologies that make coaching easier and more effective. We will continue to take leadership roles in the evolution of standards and credentialing for wellness coaches. We will continue to integrate what we know from the field of wellness and health promotion into the process of wellness coaching.

The concept of allies is central to coaching, and to wellness. We've discovered through experience and through hard evidence that connectedness is a key to lasting lifestyle improvement. We want to continue to grow this concept and find new ways to create Allies For A Healthy World.

Everyone has a stake in wellness. Being as healthy and well as possible, maximizing human potential is not just for those privileged by wealth or social status. It is for all. For those struggling economically every sick day lost at work is a threat. For those around the world in less-developed countries, what the World Health Organization calls "lifestyle diseases" are now their greatest health threat.

We will continue to rely on research and science to help us unravel the perplexing questions around the tremendous rise in obesity, diabetes, etc. We will continue to discover what todays lead pipes are. Remember how the Romans during the days of their great empire used lead pipes for their public water supply? There may be things we take for granted today that are slowly "poisoning" us as well.

As we wait for the evidence to arrive we need to take action on what we know works. Part of that comes from behavioral science, not just chemistry and biology. Wellness coaching needs to continue to ground itself in the best of behavioral science. We need to continually balance this information and these concepts with the compassion and love that we have for our fellow human beings and the world around us. Staying true to the foundational principles of coaching can help us do that.

Thirty five years of professional involvement in the wellness field has taught me that wellness is about personal growth and it's currency is connectedness. It's tempting to make wellness all about the statistics. Biometric markers are easy to measure. Cost savings are a great bottom line. Healthcare has become a business. We need to continually ask ourselves as we present to another human being, someone seeking to improve their way of living, seeking to improve their health… "Are we following a path with heart?"

> *"For me there is only the traveling on the paths that have heart, on any path that may have heart. There I travel, and the only worthwhile challenge for me is to traverse its full length. And there I travel—looking, looking, breathlessly."*

Carlos Castaneda
from *The Teachings of Don Juan: A Yaqui Way Of Knowledge*

Post Script

My own wellness journey, like that of most of us, has included many twists and turns. The day after I sent the first draft of the manuscript for this book to my editor, I left to keynote on wellness coaching in London. The keynote and workshop were very well received, but the next day I seemed to be coming down with a severe chest cold. A couple of days later, as we began some touring, a doctor in Wales told me that yes, I probably had an upper respiratory infection, and by the way, had anyone ever told me that I had a heart murmur? My stamina diminished day by day and soon I was in a hospital emergency ward having difficulty breathing. Six days in a British hospital and the conclusion was finally reached that my mitral valve had sprung loose and blood was backing up into the upper chamber. My lungs were filling with fluid.

I managed to return home to Colorado and have the surgery there as I began going into congestive heart failure. When they did a heart catheterization the day before surgery, the technician told me that my arteries were clean as a whistle! No heart disease at all. All that good wellness lifestyle effort had not been in vain!

In earlier years I had been through other major surgeries. With all of this behind me I thought I knew what surgery felt like. Open heart surgery is a whole different experience, it's more like a train wreck.

While not as common as bypass surgery, valve surgery is just as severe, and sometimes more so. The chest is opened by splitting the sternum and the wall of the heart is sliced into. I was very fortunate. I had no heart disease. I had no diabetes. I was in very good physical condition to start with…and, instead of valve replacement, my gifted surgeon was able to repair the existing valve.

As I lay in my hospital bed with a view of the Front Range foothills, a nurse began saying how my good physical condition had been a distinct advantage for me. I asked her to look out the window at Greyrock Mountain on the Rocky Mountain skyline. "You see Greyrock? A month ago I climbed that." She was astonished. We both paused and reflected on the unpredictability of life. Now, months later, after weeks in cardiac rehabilitation, and tremendous support from my wife Deborah, friends and family, I am recuperating well and on the way back to good health.

I've always been a believer in experiential education, but this may have been taking it too far! I have had great ability to empathize with another's experience, but what an intimate and total way to know what major health challenges are really all about! The powerful experiences of the last year have taught me many things on a deeper level than before: Patience, faith, tenacity, and the importance of connectedness.

I've seen myself go from where the distance from bed to bathroom was a challenge, to where walking around the block was a daunting task, to where I'm walking all-day hikes with great stamina. I've gone from a weight lifting limit of less than five pounds to where I'm pressing over seventy pounds on a chest press. Working out in cardiac rehab while the speakers played Van Halen and Santana was something I had never envisioned!

More than anything, though, I am so thankful I didn't have to go through this experience alone. That is one thing I can't imagine, and would not wish for anyone. "Connection is the currency of wellness," is what my friend Jack Travis likes to say. Lack of it has to be the worst kind of impoverishment.

In the British hospital I shared a wardroom with five other men. One was bedridden, three could sit beside their beds only, and another chap and I were able to walk about for short distances. It was like a scene from *The English Patient,* or *For Whom The Bell Tolls*. In the bed beside me, a kind, but tough, old fellow was battling emphysema with bulldog determination, swearing that he'd danced with the devil a few times, but he wasn't going to get him yet! Across the way, the bedridden man, who was deaf and mute, was visited everyday by family members who signed to him and did what they could. All around me nurses, nurses aids, cleaning ladies, and doctors showed the most amazing compassion and dedication.

As I watched the men of the ward, I thought of those Hemingway-type scenes and how we justly honor the soldiers who have been wounded, as heroes. No less heroic are the efforts of all of these men, their families, the staff, medical and optherwise, who care for them around the world. The patients summon the courage to sit up, to draw deep for that breath, and to heal as they are able. Their caregivers look past the things that would frighten and repel, or at least discourage, many of us, past the smells, the messes, and the expressions of pain, to connect with this fellow human in front of them and show them love.

I was given inspiration by the tenderness, mercy, strength and courage I saw on that ward, and in my own Colorado hospital. I was reminded of the many expressions of caring and connection shown to me, my loved ones and others throughout my life. In hospitals, funeral homes, schools, counseling centers, and treatment facilities of all kinds, and in day-to-day life, wherever that acknowledgement is made that we were all given to each other to help one another, we see the power of connection.

Appendix I
Coaching Core Competencies*

The following eleven core coaching competencies were developed to support greater understanding about the skills and approaches used within today's coaching profession as defined by the International Coaching Federation (ICF). They will also support you in calibrating the level of alignment between the coach-specific training expected and the training you have experienced.

These competencies were used as the foundation for the ICF Credentialing process examination. The core competencies are grouped into four clusters according to those that fit together logically based on common ways of looking at the competencies in each group. The groupings and individual competencies are not weighted—they do not represent any kind of priority in that they are all core or critical for any competent coach to demonstrate.

A. Setting the Foundation

1. Meeting Ethical Guidelines and Professional Standards—
Ability to understand coaching ethics and standards to apply them appropriately in all coaching situations

   a. Understands and exhibits in own behaviors the ICF Standards of Conduct (see list)

   b. Understands and follows all ICF Ethical Guidelines (see list)

   c. Clearly communicates the distinctions between coaching, consulting, psychotherapy, and other support professions

   d. Refers client to another support professional as needed, knowing when this is needed and the available resources

2. Establishing the Coaching Agreement—
Ability to understand what is required in the specific coaching

---

*Taken from the International Coaching Fereration's *Professional Coaching Core Competencies*

interaction and to come to agreement with the prospective and new client about the coaching process and relationship

   a. Understands and effectively discusses with the client the guidelines and specific parameters of the coaching relationship (e.g., logistics, fees, scheduling, inclusion of others if appropriate)

   b. Reaches agreement about what is appropriate in the relationship and what is not, what is and is not being offered, and about the client's and coach's responsibilities

   c. Determines whether there is an effective match between his/her coaching method and the needs of the prospective client

B. Co-Creating the Relationship

3. Establishing Trust and Intimacy with the Client—

Ability to create a safe, supportive environment that produces ongoing mutual respect and trust

   a. Shows genuine concern for the client's welfare and future

   b. Continuously demonstrates personal integrity, honesty, and sincerity

   c. Establishes clear agreements and keeps promises

   d. Demonstrates respect for client's perceptions, learning style, personal being

   e. Provides ongoing support for and champions new behaviors and actions, including those involving risk taking and fear of failure

   f. Asks permission to coach client in sensitive, new areas

4. Coaching Presence—

Ability to be fully conscious of and to create spontaneous

relationship with the client, employing a style that is open, flexible and confident

   a. Is present and flexible during the coaching process, dancing in the moment

   b. Accesses own intuition and trusts one's inner knowing — goes with the gut

   c. Is open to not knowing and willing to take risks

   d. Sees many ways to work with the client, and chooses what is most effective in the moment

   e. Uses humor effectively to create lightness and energy

   f. Confidently shifts perspectives and experiments with new possibilities for own action

   g. Demonstrates confidence in working with strong emotions; can self-manage and not be overpowered or enmeshed by client's emotions.

C. Communicating Effectively

5. Active Listening—

Ability to focus completely on what the client is saying or is not saying, to understand the meaning of what is said in the context of the client's desires, and to support client self-expression

   a. Attends to the client and the client's agenda, and not to the coach's agenda for the client

   b. Hears the client's concerns, goals, values, and beliefs about what is and is not possible

   c. Distinguishes between the words, the tone of voice, and the body language

   d. Summarizes, paraphrases, reiterates, mirrors back what client has said to ensure clarity and understanding

e. Encourages, accepts, explores and reinforces the client's expression of feelings, perceptions, concerns, beliefs, suggestions, etc.

f. Integrates and builds on client's ideas and suggestions

g. Bottom-lines or understands the essence of the client's communication and helps the client get there rather than engaging in long descriptive stories

h. Allows the client to vent or clear the situation without judgment or attachment in order to move on to next steps

6. Powerful Questioning —

Ability to ask questions that reveal the information needed for maximum benefit to the coaching relationship and the client

a. Asks questions that reflect active listening and an understanding of the client's perspective

b. Asks questions that evoke discovery, insight, commitment or action (e.g., those that challenge the client's assumptions)

c. Asks open-ended questions that create greater clarity, possibility, or new learning direction. Asks questions that move the client towards what they desire, not questions that ask for the client to justify or look backwards

7. Direct Communication —

Ability to communicate effectively during coaching sessions, and to use language that has the greatest positive impact on the client

a. Is clear, articulate, and direct in sharing and providing feedback

b. Reframes and articulates to help the client understand from another perspective what he/she wants or is uncertain about

c. Clearly states coaching objectives, meeting agenda, purpose of techniques or exercises

d. Uses language appropriate and respectful to the client (e.g., non-sexist, non-racist, non-technical, non-jargon)

e. Uses metaphor and analogy to help to illustrate a point or paint a verbal picture

D. Facilitating Learning and Results

8. Creating Awareness—
Ability to integrate and accurately evaluate multiple sources of information, and to make interpretations that help the client to gain awareness and thereby achieve agreed-upon results

a. Goes beyond what is said in assessing client's concerns, not getting hooked by the client's description

b. Invokes inquiry for greater understanding, awareness and clarity

c. Identifies for the client his/her underlying concerns, typical and fixed ways of perceiving himself/herself and the world, differences between the facts and the interpretation, disparities between thoughts, feelings and action

d. Helps clients to discover for themselves the new thoughts, beliefs, perceptions, emotions, moods, etc. that strengthen their ability to take action and achieve what is important to them

e. Communicates broader perspectives to clients and inspires commitment to shift their viewpoints and find new possibilities for action

f Helps clients to see the different, interrelated factors that affect them and their behaviors (e.g., thoughts, emotions, body, background)

285

g. Expresses insights to clients in ways that are useful and meaningful for the client

h. Identifies major strengths vs. major areas for learning and growth, and what is most important to address during coaching

i. Asks the client to distinguish between trivial and significant issues, situational vs. recurring behaviors, when detecting a separation between what is being stated and what is being done

9. Designing Actions—

Ability to create with the client opportunities for ongoing learning, during coaching, and in work/life situations, and for taking new actions that will most effectively lead to agreed-upon coaching results

a. Brainstorms and assists the client to define actions that will enable the client to demonstrate, practice and deepen new learning,

b. Helps the client to focus on and systematically explore specific concerns and opportunities that are central to agreed-upon coaching goals,

c. Engages the client to explore alternative ideas and solutions, to evaluate options, and to make related decisions,

d. Promotes active experimentation and self-discovery, to facilitate the client's ability to apply what has been discussed and learned during sessions immediately afterwards in his/her work or life setting,

e. Celebrates client successes and capabilities for future growth

f. Challenges client's assumptions and perspectives to provoke new ideas and find new possibilities for action

g. Advocates or brings forward points of view that are aligned with client goals and, without attachment, engages the client to consider them

h. Helps the client "Do It Now" during the coaching session, providing immediate support

i. Encourages, stretches, and challenges client's learning pace while recognizing and accepting their comfort level

10. Planning and Goal Setting—

Ability to develop and maintain an effective coaching plan with the client

a. Consolidates collected information and establishes a coaching plan and development of goals with the client that address concerns and major areas for learning and development

b. Creates a plan with results that are attainable, measurable, specific, and have target dates

c. Makes plan adjustments as warranted by the coaching process and by changes in the situation

d. Helps the client identify and access different resources for learning (e.g., books, other professionals)

e. Identifies and targets early successes that are important to the client

11. Managing Progress and Accountability—

Ability to hold attention on what is important for the client, and to leave responsibility with the client to take action

a. Clearly requests client actions that will move the client toward their stated goals

b. Demonstrates follow through by asking the client about those actions that the client committed to during the previous session(s)

287

c. Acknowledges the client for what they have done, not done, learned or become aware of since the previous coaching session(s)

d. Effectively prepares, organizes, and reviews information obtained during sessions with client

e. Keeps the client on track between sessions by focusing attention on the coaching plan and outcomes, agreed-upon courses of action, and topics for future session(s)

f. Focuses on the coaching plan while being open to adjusting behaviors and actions based on the coaching process and shifts in direction during sessions

g. Moves back and forth between the big picture of where the client is heading, setting a context for what is being discussed, where the client wishes to go, and where the client is at that session

h. Promotes client's self-discipline and holds the client accountable for what they say they are going to do, for the results of an intended action, or for a specific plan with related time frames

i. Develops the client's ability to make decisions, address key concerns, and develop himself/herself (to get feedback, to determine priorities, and set the pace of learning, to reflect on and learn from experiences)

j. Positively confronts the client when he/she did not take agreed-upon actions

Appendix II
Wellness Mapping 360° Welcome Packet

Personal Information

(Completely confidential)

LAST NAME _____

FIRST NAME _____

NAME YOU LIKE TO BE CALLED _____

MAILING ADDRESS

    STREET, RR, ETC. _____

    CITY _____ STATE _____

    ZIP CODE _____ COUNTRY _____

PHONE INFO *(Please put a check mark by the phone # you want to be primarily called at)*

    HOME TELEPHONE (_____) _____

    WORK TELEPHONE (_____) _____

    MESSAGE OR MOBILE PHONE (_____) _____

    FAX NUMBER (_____) _____

E-MAIL ADDRESS _____

OCCUPATION/NATURE OF BUSINESS_____

_____

EMPLOYER NAME (OR NAME OF YOUR BUSINESS) _____

ADDRESS OF SAME _____

DATE OF BIRTH _____ MARITAL STATUS _____

SIGNIFICANT OTHERS NAME _____

NAME(S) OF CHILD(REN)/STEPCHILD(REN) AND THEIR AGE(S) (LIST BELOW AND ON BACK IF NEEDED)

_____

289

Please write a brief description of:

Your Education History: colleges attended, degrees, majors, etc., other trainings.

_____

_____

_____

_____

_____

Your Work History: basics of the type of work/career areas you have experienced, and for how long.

_____

_____

_____

_____

_____

Your Relationship History: chronicle your marriage(s), long-term relationships, etc.

_____

_____

_____

_____

_____

Thank you very much! This information helps me be the very best coach for you!

Focusing Your Choices

An aspect of the coaching process is to assist you in clarifying your direction in your life style choices. This exercise will add clarity to the primary areas you want to focus on in coaching. Please describe the five areas you would like to change or improve in your way of living. How will it look when you accomplish your goals?

1. What I would like to change or improve is . . .

_____

_____

How will your life/health change when this is improved or changed?

_____

_____

2. What I would like to change or improve is . . .

_____

_____

How will your life/health change when this is improved or changed?

_____

_____

3. What I would like to change or improve is . . .

_____

_____

How will your life/health change when this is improved or changed?

_____

_____

4. What I would like to change or improve is . . .

_____

_____

How will your life/health change when this is improved or changed?

_____

_____

5. What I would like to change or improve is . . .

_____

_____

How will your life/health change when this is improved or changed?

_____

_____

10 Things You Want Me to Know About You

1. _____
_____
_____

2. _____
_____
_____

3. _____
_____
_____

4. _____
_____
_____

5. _____
_____
_____

6. _____
_____
_____

7. _____
_____
_____

8. _____
_____
_____

9. _____
_____
_____

10. _____
_____

Laying the Foundation for Coaching

As your coach, it's important for me to understand how you view the world in general, yourself, your family and your job or career. Each person comes from a unique place in their thinking and their interaction with the world around them.

Answering these questions clearly and thoughtfully, will serve both you and me. The questions may help you clarify perceptions about yourself and the direction of your life. These are "pondering" type questions, designed to stimulate your thinking in a way that will make our work together more productive. Take your time answering them. If they are not complete by our first (foundation) session, bring what you have completed and finish the rest later. These answers will be treated with complete professional confidentiality.

Occupation / nature of business: _____

_____

Employers or Business Name: _____

Date of birth: _____ Marital status: _____

Do you have children? _____

Do your children live with you? _____

Coaching

1. What do want to get from the coaching relationship?

_____

_____

2. What is the best way for me to coach you most effectively, what tips would you give to me about what would work best?

_____

_____

3. Do you have any apprehension or preconceived ideas of coaching?

_____

_____

Job/Career

1. What do you want from your job/career?

_____

_____

2. What projects or tasks are you involved in currently or regularly?

_____

_____

3. What are your key job/career goals currently?

_____

_____

4. What skills or knowledge are you developing? How are you gaining this knowledge?

_____

_____

5. How do your job/career goals support or fit with your personal goals or sense of purpose?

_____

_____

6. In what ways does your job affect your level of stress and your health?

_____

_____

Personal

1. What accomplishments or events must, in your opinion, occur during your lifetime to consider your life satisfying and well-lived?

_____

_____

2. What is (or might be) a secret passion in your life? Something you may or may not have allowed yourself to do so far, but you would really love to do.

_____

_____

3. What unique gift or knowledge do you have to contribute?

_____

_____

4. What is your spiritual base or belief system? How do your draw upon your spiritual beliefs for support and to help you with moving forward with your life?

_____

_____

5. Please describe what gives you a sense of purpose in life? What activities have meaning or heart for you?

_____

_____

6. What's missing in your life, the presence of which would make your life be more fulfilling?

_____

_____

7. What do you do when you are really stressed, and feel up against the wall?

_____

_____

8. What two steps could you take immediately that would make the greatest difference in your current situation?

_____

_____

9. What else would you like your coach to know about you?

_____

_____

Health & Wellness Information

As your coach, my job is not to treat you, but to be your ally and your resource. When it comes to health and wellness issues I will help you discover steps you may choose to take towards greater health and higher levels of wellness.

As your ally, I may refer you to medical, psychological, nutritional and other health-related services for more information and to seek treatment in these areas. I can be a source of support and accountability, helping you to follow through with any treatment plans that you devise with these other professionals.

Please share with me information about your health and wellness so that I may more fully understand your health challenges and aspirations for higher levels of wellness.

1. Please describe your lifestyle and what you do to be healthy and well.

_____

_____

2. Please describe any health challenges that you currently experience (including not only major concerns, but problems like headaches, insomnia, etc.)

_____

_____

3. Are you currently on any medications? If so what is the name of the medication and the intended impact of the medication?

_____

_____

4. Please list any lifestyle changes/recommendations that have recently been made to you by a healthcare professional.

_____

_____

5. What do you do to reduce stress in your life, or to counter-act the effect of stress in your life?

_____

_____

6. Please describe a typical week in terms of diet and exercise.

_____

_____

7. What do you do in your life that brings you happiness and joy? How often do you do this?

_____

_____

8. What gets in the way of you doing what brings you joy and health in the world?

_____

_____

9. Please list the behaviors you'd like to change and then rate your readiness to make changes on each of the identified behaviors you listed.

    1 = Haven't even thought of changing this

    2 = Have given it some thought

    3 = Have started preparing to change (have looked up information, talked with others about it, etc.)

    4 = Am already taking some action to change in this area

    5 = Have already made the change and want help maintaining my progress

WHAT BEHAVIORS RELATED TO YOUR LIFE STYLE DO YOU WANT TO CHANGE?	RATE READI-NESS 1–5	COMMENTS

10. How can a coach be of assistance in helping you make the lifestyle changes you'd like to make?

_____

_____

11. What else would you like to add about your wellness goals?

_____

_____

Please take the time to think about the different areas of your life reflected in the Wheel of Life Below. Rate yourself in each category.

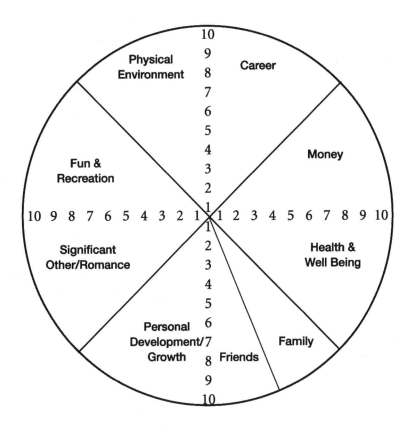

The nine sections in the Wheel of Life represent fulfillment and balance. Rank your level of satisfaction in each life area by marking the number and drawing a line in each section to create a new outer edge of the wheel. The closer you are to a 10, the more fulfilled you are. The new perimeter of the circle you draw represents your Wheel of Life. How bumpy would the ride be if this were a real wheel? "The Wheel of Life", a simple pie chart, is a commonly used tool in the health and wellness fields and is public domain property. Please copy it, and use it.

Bibliography & Resources

Ardell, Donald. (1996) *The Book of Wellness: A Secular Approach to Spirit, Meaning & Purpose*. Amherst, NY: Prometheus Books.

Ardell, Donald. (1982) *14 Days To A Wellness Lifestyle*. Mill Valley, CA: Whatever Publishing, Inc.

Ardell, D.B. (1986) *High Level Wellness: An Alternative to Doctors, Drugs and Disease. 10th Anniversary Ed.* Berkeley, CA: Ten Speed Press.

Arloski, M. (2013) "How To Influence Lasting Lifestyle Change: The Benefits of Wellness Coaching – Parts One and Two of an Interview with Dr. Michael Arloski On The Art & Science of Coaching." WELCOA's News & Views – Expert Interview Series. http://welcoa.org/freeresources/index.php?category=16

Arloski, M. (2010) *Your Journey To A Healthier Life: Paths of Wellness Guided Journal, Vol. One*. Duluth, MN: Whole Person Associates.

Arloski, M. (2008) "Wellness Coaching and Lifestyle Medicine: Covering The Whole Continuum." *Wellness Management,* The National Wellness Institute, September 2008.

Arloski, M. (2006) "New Mindset, New Model: From Prescribe and Treat, or Educate and Implore, to Advocate and Inspire - The Coach Approach!"

Coach (Magazine of Coaching & Mentoring International), March/April, 2006

Arloski, M. (2004) The Wellness Coach: Lifestyle Prescriptions Filled Here. *Tomorrow's Life Coach*, Institute For Life Coach Training. Volume 3 Issue 1 :January 2004.

Arloski, M. (2003) "Lasting Lifestyle Change Through Wellness Coaching." *Wellness Management*, Spring 2003.

Arloski, M. (2002) "Simply Centered" Unpublished document. Available through the author. Also available at the author's website: www.realbalance.com

Arloski, M. (2002) "The Power of Habit" Unpublished document. Available through the author. Also available at the author's website: www.realbalance.com

Arloski, M. (1999) "Coaching For Wellness." *Wellness Management,* The National Wellness Institute, Winter 1999.

Arloski, M. (1994) "The Ten Tenets of Wellness." *Wellness Management,*

Carson, Rick. (2003) *Taming Your Gremlin: A Surprisingly Simple Method for Getting Out of Your Own Way, Rev. Ed.* New York: Quill/Harper Collins.

Cashman, Kevin. (2000) *Leadership From The Inside Out: Becoming A Leader for Life.* Provo, UT: Executive Excellence Publishing.

Chapman, Larry, S. (2013) "Nine Reasons Why Wellness Works" January 04, 2013 CFO.com I US

Chapman, Larry S., Lesch, N., Baun, M.P. (2007) "The role of health and wellness coaching in worksite health promotion." *American Journal of Health Promotion*, Vol. 21, No. 6. (2007) Key: citeulike:5010209

Chapman, Larry. (2002) *Proof Positive: The Practitioner's Guide To ROI and Program Development*, Edition #5, Summex Health Management. Retrieved from WELCOA: http://www.welcoa. org/store/ML0002.html

Chodron, Pema. (2000) *When Things Fall Apart: Heart Advice for Difficult Times.* Boston, London: Shambhala Classics.

Covey, Stephen. (1989) *The Seven Habits of Highly Effective People.* New York: Simon & Schuester, Inc.

"The Coaching Connection – Special Edition" of *Absolute Advantage: The Workplace Wellness Magazine.* The Wellness Councils of America. 2002, 1/10.

Crum, Thomas. (1987) *The Magic of Conflict: Turning A Life of Work Into A Work of Art.* New York: Touchstone/Simon & Schuster, Inc.

Czimbal, Bob & Zadikov, Maggie (2005) *Kindred Spirits: The Quest for Love and Friendship.* Portland, OR: Open Book Publishers & The Abundance Co.

Czimbal, Bob & Zadikov, Maggie (1999) *Vitamin T - A Guide to Healthy Touch.* Portland, OR: The Abundance Co.

de Lorgeril M, Salen P, Martin JL, et al. Mediterranean diet, traditional risk factors, and the rate of cardiovascular complications after myocardial infarction: final report of the Lyon Diet Heart Study. *Circulation.* 99:779–785.

Donaldson, O. Fred. (1993) *Playing By Heart: The Vision and Practice of Belonging.* Deerfield Beach, FL: Health Communications, Inc.

Edelman D, Oddone,E, Liebowitz RS, Yancy WS, Olsen MK, Jeffreys AS, Moon SD, Harris AC, Smith LL, Quillian-Wolever R, Gaudet TW. (2006) "A Multidimensional Integrative Medicine Intervention to Improve Cardiovascular Risk." *Journal of General Internal Medicine,* 21/7, 728–734.

Ellis, Dave. (1998) *Life Coaching: A New Career for Helping Professionals.* Rapid City, SD: Breakthrough Enterprises.

Ellis, Dave. (2000) *Falling Awake.* Rapid City, SD: Breakthrough Enterprises.

Flaherty, James. (1999) *Coaching: Evoking Excellence in Others.* Boston: Butterworth & Heinemann.

Giesen, Greg. (2003) *Creating Authenticity: Meaningful Questions for the Minds & Souls of Today's Leaders.* Denver, CO: GGA, Inc. Publishers.

Hargrove, R. (1995) *Masterful Coaching.* San Diego: Pfeiffer.

Health Promotion Practitioner (2004), Sept./Oct., 5-7. "Spotlight On Wellness Coaching: A Positive Focus For Empowering Participants." Interview with Dr. Michael Arloski and Beth Shepard.

Jampolsky, G., (1989, 2004) *Love Is Letting Go of Fear.* (25th Anniversary Ed.) Berkley/Toronto: Celestial Arts.

Kimiecik, Jay. (2002) *The Intrinsic Exerciser: Discovering the Joy of Exercise.* Boston, New York: Houghton Mifflin Co.

Kimsey-House, H., Sandahl, P., Whitworth, L. (2011) *Co-Active Coaching: Changing Business, Transforming Lives. 3rd Ed.,* Palo Alto, CA: Davies-Black.

Lambert, Michael J., Barley, Dean E. (2001) "Research Summary on the Therapeutic Relationship and Psychotherapy Outcome." *Psychotherapy: Theory, Research, Practice, Training*, Vol 38(4), Win, 357-361. doi: 10.1037/0033-3204.38.4.357

Leonard, Thomas. (1998) *The Portable Coach: 28 Surefire Strategies for Business and Personal Success*. New York: Scribner.

Levine, James A. (2009) *Move A Little, Lose A Lot*. Crown Publisher, New York.

Levine, Stephen. (1989) *Who Dies? An Investigation of Conscious Living and conscious Dying*. New York: Doubleday.

Lowery, S. & Menendez, D. (1997) *Discovering Your Best Self Through The Art of Coaching*. Houston: Nexus Point/Enterprise.

Lusk, Julie. (1992) *30 Scripts For Relaxation, Imagery & Inner Healing*. Duluth, MN: Whole Person Associates.

Lusk, Julie. (1993) *30 Scripts For Relaxation, Imagery & Inner Healing, Volume II*. Duluth, MN: Whole Person Associates.

Lusk, Julie. (1998) *Desktop Yoga: The Anytime, Anywhere Relaxation Program for Office Slaves, Internet Addicts, and Stressed-Out Students*. New York: Perigee.

Lynn Smith-Lovin with Miller McPherson & Matthew Brashears (2006) "Social Isolation in America: Changes in Core Discussion Networks over Two Decades." *American Sociological Review* 71:3.

Maslow, Abraham. (1962) *Toward A Psychology of Being*. Princeton, NJ: Van Nostrand.

Miller, W.R. & Rollnick, S. (2002) *Motivational Interviewing, 2nd Ed.: Preparing People for Change*. New York: Gullford Press.

Moore, M. & Tschannen-Moran, R. (2009) *Coaching Psychology Manual*. Lippincott Williams & Wilkins.

Moore, Thomas. (1992) *Care of The Soul: A Guide for Cultivating Depth and Sacredness in Everyday Life*. New York: Harper Perennial.

Nepo, Mark. (2000) *The Book of Awakening: Having the Life You Want by Being Present to the Life You Have*. Newburyport, MA: Conari Press.

Nepo, Mark. (2007) *Facing the Lion, Being the Lion: Finding Inner Courage Where It Lives*. Newburyport, MA: Conari Press.

Ornish, D. et al (1990). "Can lifestyle changes reverse coronary heart disease?" The Lifestyle Heart Trial. Lancet Jul 21, 336(8708), 129-33

Ornish, D. (2002) Intensive lifestyle changes in management of coronary heart disease. *Harrison's Advances in Cardiology*. Edited by E. Braunwald. New York: McGraw-Hill, 2002

Patterson, K., Grenny, J., McMillian, R. & Switzler, A. (2002) *Crucial Conversations: Tools for Talking When Stakes Are High*. New York: McGraw-Hill.

Phillips, Bill. (1999) *Body for Life: 12 Weeks to Mental and Physical Strength*. New York: Harper Collins.

Pink, Daniel. (2010) *Drive: The Surprising Truth About What Motivates Us*. Edinburgh: Canongate.

Prochaska, J., Norcross, J, & Diclemente, C. (1994) *Changing For Good*. New York: Harper Collins/Quill.

Pilzer, P.Z. (2007) *The Wellness Revolution*. Hoboken, NJ: John Wiley & Sons.

Putnam, R.D. (2001) *Bowling Alone: The Collapse and Revival of American Community*. New York: Simon & Schuster.

Richardson, C. (1998) *Take Time For Your Life: A Personal Coach's Seven Step Program for Creating The Life You Want*. New York: Broadway.

Ruiz, D.M. (1997) *The Four Agreements: A Toltec Wisdom Book*. San Rafael, CA: Amber-Allen Publishing, Inc.

Seaward, B.L. (1997) *Managing Stress: Principles and Strategies for Health and Wellbeing. 2nd Ed.* Sudbury, MA: Jones and Bartlett Publishers.

Schwartz, T., et. al. (2010) *The Way We're Working Isn't Working*. New York: Free Press.

"Spotlight On Wellness Coaching: A Positive Focus For Empowering Participants." Interview with Dr. Michael Arloski and Beth Shepard. (2004) *Health Promotion Practitioner*, Sept./Oct., Vol. 13, Issue 5, 5-7.

Travis, J.W. & Ryan, R.S. (2004) *Wellness Workbook: How To Achieve Enduring Heatlh and Vitality, 3ʳᵈ Ed*. Berkeley, Toronto: Celestial Arts.

Vale MJ, Jelinek MV, Best JD, Dart AM, Grigg LE, Hare DL, Ho BP, Newman RW, & McNeil JJ; (2003) Coaching Patients on Achieving Cardiovascular Health (COACH): A Multicenter Randomized Trial in Patients with Coronary Heart Disease. *Archives of Internal Medicine*. Dec 8-22;163(22):2775-83.

Watson, Jeanne C. "Reassessing Rogers' Necessary and Sufficient Conditions of Change." *Psychotherapy: Theory, Research, Practice, Training*, Vol 44(3), Sep 2007, 268-273.

Whitmore, J. (1995) *Coaching for Performance*. Sonoma, CA: Nicholas Brealey.

Williams, P. & Menendez, D. (2007) *Becoming a Professional Life Coach: Lessons from the Institute for Life Coach Training*. New York: W.W. Norton & Co.

Williams, P. & Anderson, S.K. (2006) *Law & Ethics in Coaching: How to Solve and Avoid Difficult Problems in Your Practice*. Hoboken, NJ: John Wiley & Sons, Inc.

Williams, P. (2004) "Coaching and the Wellness Industry: A New Gateway for Consumer Awareness." *Choice*, vol. 2, issue 2.

Williams, P. & Thomas, L. *Total Life Coaching: A Compendium Of Resources*. New York: W.W. Norton & Co.

Williams, P. & Davis, D.C. (2002) *Therapist as Life Coach: Transforming Your Practice*. New York: W.W. Norton & Co.

Wolever, R. Q., Dreusicke, M.H., Fikkan, J.L., Hawkins, T.V., Yeung, S.Y., Wakefield, J., Duda, L., Flowers, P., Cook, C., & Skinner, E. (2010) "Integrative Health Coaching for Patients with Type 2 Diabetes: A Randomized Clinical Trial." *Diabetes Educator, 36(4), doi* . 10.1177/0145721710371523.

Wolever, R.Q., Webber, D.M., Meunier, J.P., Greeson, J. M., Lausier, E.R., & Gaudet, T.W. (In press). "Modifiable Disease Risk, Readiness to Change, and Psychosocial Functioning Improve with Integrative Medicine Immersion Model." *Alternative Therapies in Health and Medicine*.

References

Institutes & Organizations

American Cancer Society:
www.cancer.org

American Diabetes Association:
www.diabetes.org

American Heart Association: Cholesterol levels:
www.americanheart.org

American Holistic Health Association:
www.ahha.org

The Institute For Life Coach Training.
www.lifecoachtraining.com

The International Coaches Federation.
www.coachfederation.org

National Wellness Institute/Conference
www.nationalwellness.org

National Consortium For Credentialing Health & Wellness Coaches
www.ncchwc.org

Real Balance Global Wellness Services, Inc.
www.realbalance.com

Wellcoaches Corporation
www.wellcoaches.com

Good Web References

Abundance Company/Bob Czimbal: Great handouts on wellness, humor and connectedness.
www.abundancecompany.com/free_handouts.htm

Body For Life: Fitness and diet program:
www.bodyforlife.com

E-diets - Central clearing house for online diets and diet services:
www.ediets.com/index.cfm

HealthWorld Online: Endless wellness/health information, articles, speakers, and medline searches: (Jim Strohecker & The Wellness Inventory)
www.healthy.net

My Food Diary - subscriber-based online food journal, etc.:
www.myfooddiary.com

OncoLink large web resource on cancer:
www.oncolink.upenn.edu/types/

PubMed - The National Library of Medicine/National Institutes of Health - great resource for journal articles, etc.:
www.ncbi.nlm.nih.gov/entrez/query.fcgi?db=PubMed

Real Age - Simple, free, online HRA type instrument
www.realage.com

Sacred Passage and The Way of Nature Fellowship/John P. Milton: Contemporary Vision Quests, Meditation Retreats, Qi Gong and T'ai Chi Training, Study of ancient Shamanic Practices, and Traditional Wilderness Vision Quests:
www.sacredpassage.com/

Whole Person Associates: Publishers of a wide variety of wellness and stress management books, tools and resources:
www.wholeperson.com

The Wellness Inventory:
www.mywellnesstest.com

Wholesome Resources/Julie Lusk: Yoga, Meditation, Guided Imagery, Affirmations, Stress Relief and Wellness:
www.relaxationstation.com

Fitness & Wellness Apps

www.sportypal.com
www.fitday.com
myfitnesspal.com
loseit.com
fatsecret.com
everydayhealth.com/
    my-calorie-counter
caloriecount.about.com

onlinefitnesslog.com
fitwatch.com/diary/
livestrong.com/thedailyplate/
fitclick.com
mapmywalk.com
gmap-pedometer.com
mapmyrun.com
prevention.com/mywalkingmaps/

Training and Certification in
Wellness & Health Coaching

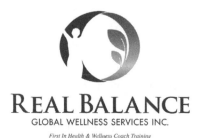

REAL BALANCE
GLOBAL WELLNESS SERVICES INC.

First In Health & Wellness Coach Training

Real Balance Global Wellness Services, Inc.
The Wellness Coach Training Institute
www.realbalance.com

The author, Dr. Arloski, is the founder and CEO of Real Balance Global Wellness Services, Inc. His company has trained thousands of health & wellness coaches worldwide. Their coursework is approved for ACSTH – Approved Coach Specific Training Hours – by the International Coaching Federation (ICF). It is also approved by The American College of Sports Medicine (ACSM), The American Holistic Nurses Association (AHNA), The National Commission for Health Education Credentialing, Inc. (CHES), and other credentialing bodies for continuing education credit for these professions and for P.A.'s, P.T.'s, and others. Real Balance Coach Certification Training is offered live and via live, interactive webinars worldwide. For complete information visit www.realbalance.com, email wellness@realbalance. com, or call 1-866-568-4702.

Follow Dr. Arloski's Blog

For In-depth articles on wellness & wellness coaching

Wellness Wisdom And Wanderings
http://realbalancewellness.wordpress.com

Your Journey To A Healthier Life:
Paths of Wellness Guided Journal, Vol. 1.

The worksheets and handouts conrtained in this book are available from the publisher in CD format:

Whole Person Associates, Duluth, MN
800-247-6789, www.wholeperson.com

Also available by Michael Arloski . . .

Your Journey to a Healthier Life

MICHAEL ARLOSKI, PHD, PCC

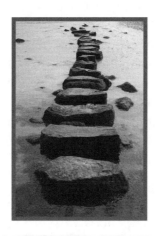

WHOLE PERSON ASSOCIATES

DULUTH, MINNESOTA

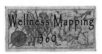
THE JOURNEY BEGINS . . .

Think of this guided wellness journal as a tool for you to use in crafting the kind of healthy and well life that you want. Although you can use this journal on your own, the best way to work with this tool is with others through individual or group wellness coaching. My coaching colleague, Pat Williams likes to say "If you could have done it by yourself, you probably would have done it by now." Lifestyle change is much easier when we work with an ally or allies.

This guidebook will help you chart and navigate your way through the wellness coaching process and ultimately to lifestyle changes that last. Many of the tools and methods in this guide are presented in the book *Wellness Coaching For Lasting Lifestyle Change* (also by Michael Arloski). Through the work you do on your own, or with your coach or coaching group you will discover new insights about yourself and your way of living and translate them into action. This guide will provide you with ways to stay organized and on track. Think of it as a place where you can store what you need for your journey, kind of like a suitcase or backpack. It contains your map, compass, and gear for all kinds of weather and other challenges!

Remember that like any *trip* that becomes a *journey*, much of the adventure and reward is along the path, not just at the destination. Enjoy what you find along the way. Don't become so concerned with your outcome and lose your experience of the right here right now. At the same time we might say *keep your eyes on the prize*. This guide will help you do both, as will the coaching process.

Create your vision of a healthy and well life. Take stock of your life. Map out your course. Enlist the support you need. Reflect deeply. Keep track of where you are and where you are going. Acknowledge the challenges and the joys life brings.

Celebrate success! Happy traveling!

Michael Arloski, Ph.D., PCC

"The most fundamental aggression to ourselves,
the most fundamental harm we can do to ourselves,
is to remain ignorant by not having the courage
and the respect to look at ourselves
honestly and gently."

— **PEMA CHODRIN**
When Things Fall Apart

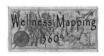

The process of change and self-exploration, insight and under-standing requires patience. Sometimes it is like the old Japanese rice farmer story. The farmer was so anxious to have his fields produce a harvest that at night he would go out and pull on the rice stalks to make them grow faster! Sometimes we too are tempted to *push the river* and realize that all we can do is be aware and find a way to ride with the current.

Taking the time to be quiet and reflective is key to the explora-tion process. Making room in your life or in a day to still your thoughts, feel your body and observe yourself is instrumental to knowing what you want and to understand your basic responses to the world around you. The important thing here is not to *work on yourself*. It is effortless effort. It is clearing the mind so that the work done later will be fresher and more focused.

Take a few quiet moments to ponder the following . . .

If your life was a novel being written by someone else and you were the main character in the story, what great strength would the writer be developing?

_____

_____

_____

_____

What great challenge would the main character be working on in his/her life?

_____

_____

_____

_____

Has your life story developed the way you had hoped?

_____

_____

_____

_____

_____

_____

_____

_____

_____

Does any deeper meaning become apparent?

_____

_____

_____

_____

_____

_____

_____

_____

_____

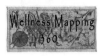

What has your physical experience been like?

_____

_____

_____

_____

_____

_____

_____

_____

_____

_____

_____

_____

_____

_____

_____

_____

_____

_____

_____

"Therefore you must always keep in mind
that a path is only a path; if you feel you should not
follow it, you must not stay with it
under any conditions...

Does this path have a heart?
If it does, the path is good; if it doesn't, it is of no use.
Both paths lead nowhere; but one has a heart,
the other doesn't. One makes for a joyful journey;
as long as you follow it, you are one with it.
The other will make you curse your life.
One makes you strong; the other weakens you."

—DON JUAN
The Teachings of Don Juan: A Yaqui Way of Knowledge by Carlos Castanada

What in your life are you grateful for?

How do you hold yourself back?

When are you at your best?

_____

_____

_____

_____

_____

_____

What brings you to wellness coaching?

_____

_____

_____

_____

_____

What are your physical concerns?

_____

_____

_____

_____

_____

_____

What were you told at your last doctors visit?

_____

_____

_____

_____

_____

_____

_____

_____

_____

_____

_____

_____

_____

_____

_____

_____

_____

_____

_____

_____

_____

_____

Whole Person Associates is the leading publisher of training resources for professionals who empower people to create and maintain healthy lifestyles. Our creative resources will help you work effectively with your clients in the areas of stress management, wellness promotion, mental health and life skills.

Please visit us at our web site: **WholePerson.com**. You can check out our entire line of products, place an order, request our print catalog, and sign up for our monthly special notifications.

Whole Person Associates
800-247-6789